Author
Leila Schwarz

Producer/coach/editor
Karin Giphart

Second editor
Phil Norris

Corrector
Hester Kuipers

Photo portrait
Imgar Libuy

Artwork back cover
Leila Schwarz

Graphic assistance
Tonio van Vugt

ISBN: 9798325954665

Published: June, 2024
Amsterdam, The Netherlands

The podcast *Lifting the Fog* by Leila Schwarz is on Spotify, Apple, and Amazon. With well-spoken and driven guests, such as Ann Cameron, the author of Curing Cancer with Carrots.

LIFTING THE FOG

How (anal) cancer improved my health and lifestyle

Leila Schwarz

This book is not intended as a substitute for medical advice of physicians. Readers should regularly consult a physician in matters relating to their health and particularly with respect to any symptoms that may require diagnosis or medical attention.

Chapters

Intro	9
1. A cancer rookie	10
2. On becoming a cancer expert	22
3. And then there was pain	35
4. The liver metastasis	38
5. Treatments	46
6. Cancer, menopause and sexuality	59
7. Cancer and work	66
8. In full remission, now what?	72
9. HPV	77
10. Cancer and family/friends	79
11. The future?	81
Acknowledgements	82
List of creams	83
Useful links	86
Glossary	94

To my wonderful family and friends
you were my rocks to hold onto in stormy weather
To my daughter
for her strength and bravery
To my love, who helped me
more than he could ever imagine
And to my little dachshund, Archimedes,
for making me walk daily.

Intro

"It has spread to the liver, which is generally not good news."

Here it is, a book I never thought I would write. A practical book on how to deal with cancer. Not just any form of cancer: anal cancer, which is a rare form of the disease but on the rise, nonetheless.
And no, I never thought I would publicly share details on such private body parts, such intimate experiences on a physical and emotional level. But, thinking about where I am now—if I were to rewind time to the moment I received the diagnosis—I'd have been grateful to find anything close to the information I'm about to share with you. It's not hard for me to talk about this chapter in my life because I believe that knowledge is key, especially at one of the most confusing times in your life.

Leila Schwarz

1. A cancer rookie

Let's get this out of the way: *anal* is a tricky word. Loaded with ridicule, shame, and prejudice. It even comes with an unwillingness to mention the very word itself. Involving the anus is all it means. The anus is an essential part of the body, unless we are Barbie or Ken, of course. It comes with all these negative associations because it is the gateway to dumping our waste.

'Being an ass' means showing some really nasty behavior.

'Being anal' means you are too controlling, very inflexible with things.

Basically, many things ass-related are not good. Unless, maybe, being a badass.

So, when dealing with anal cancer, a rare type of cancer—with numbers increasing exponentially every year—all these culturally defined sub-meanings tend to cloud any public discussion. And there are all these misconceptions, such as associating anal cancer with anal sex. And yes, infection with Human papillomavirus (HPV) can be a factor, but there are many ways in which cells can turn into cancer. Most people know very little about these topics. Neither did I.

Sharing an anal cancer diagnosis can turn into an uncomfortable conversation. Now, what would you rather tell your new boss?

A. I have colon cancer.

B. I have anal cancer.

We all know answer A raises fewer eyebrows. Some will opt for C. Not tell them at all. But you know what? I opted for B, and I'll explain why later.

First, how do you even find out if you have this particular form of cancer? There are, in fact, several forms of anal cancer. The most common type is *carcinoma*, i.e. squamous cell cancer. Squamous cells form the outer surface of organs including the anus and are also found in the vagina, cervix, bladder, urethra, and other places in the body. Another form is *adenocarcinoma* cancers which develop in the glands around the anus. Then there are skin cancers, including *basal cell* and *melanoma*, often found when they are in advanced stages.

In my case, it took many steps to get the diagnosis. Somehow, it didn't occur to me that it could be cancer. To be honest, I had never been worried about cancer. It just wasn't something in my surroundings, except for an uncle who died from cancer in 2021. He lived far away at the time. During his last years, we hardly saw one another due to distance, scheduling, and life. Though I loved my uncle dearly, I had no idea what he went through. I think it wasn't something he wanted me to be a part of, either.

When I think of my family, I feel that we are very close in many ways and share experiences outside of standard holiday celebrations. We know how to have a great time, and there are so many unforgettable parties with laughter, great conversations, and just hanging out together. However, we were never good at planning when we would see each other next or what we would do then. It is more of a spontaneous "BANG", "Wait, are we here at the same time? Let's get together!" Amazingly, this even works across large geographical distances.

Supporting each other during times of need is also something very natural in my family, though talking about and sharing significant scary situations like illnesses that could be possibly life-threatening is not natural behavior for us. Things are rather kept private, until it takes a good turn. When there is positive news, and things seem to go back to normal. So, after the fact, we tell one another.

I broke this habit.

In 2022, the week before I went on holiday, I lost a little clear blood from my bum and went to my GP about it. The suspicion was that I might have hemorrhoids, and we would follow up after the holiday. About half of the people older than 50 have hemorrhoids or piles. If you have the luxury of never experiencing piles: they are swollen veins in the rectum, sometimes external, sometimes internal. They can bleed, they are itchy, and they can be extremely painful. Women who have given birth are no strangers to them, either. So, I didn't give it another thought.

As the first half of the year had been stressful, I booked a whole month in the South of France. It was a perfect place with a terrace overlooking lush, green forest down to the coast. There was even a private swimming pool. I was a very happy bunny! In retrospect, there were some moments when I felt a little bit off; however, I couldn't pin it down to anything in particular. I did have a bit of an increased temperature at the time, multiple days, no fever really, just temperature and not for the whole day. It was a bit weird, but still nothing that would leave one really concerned. I couldn't go to the toilet during my last week in France, but even that didn't worry me. There was no pain, no nausea, no bloating.

When I came home on Saturday, things changed. In the blink of an eye, there was this belly ache that was getting worse by the minute. Considering I'd been unable to go to the bathroom, I decided that was the probable cause. I could hardly tell what kind of pain it was. It was dull and somehow pressing down. I couldn't even tell if the core of the pain was more in the front of the body or the back, which was bewildering.

On Sunday, it worsened. That indescribable feeling became unbearable. Finally, I went to the emergency pharmacy and got two mini enemas. As I stood there deciding which enema and how many to buy, I thought, this has to help, right? This has to help. Well, it was not one of my best ideas, and soon after, I called the GP's emergency number to get medical help.

They would not take me and told me I should see my GP on Monday because I wasn't nauseous. That night, the weirdest thing happened. Sleeping wasn't possible. It was more like dozing off, awake again, dozing off—until 3 AM. I got up and wanted something to drink, and after two steps, it happened: my water burst. Wait, what? I am not pregnant! I am sure of it. If you've never given birth and don't know what I'm talking about, imagine taking half a liter of water and pouring it down your legs. It was ridiculous. And it didn't stop!

Anyone who knows me will tell you that I am a logical, analytical, and pragmatic person. I mean, I work in Tech, that should tell you enough. Calmly, I tried to figure out what this could be. It felt like cellular liquid, the same stuff you find in a blister. Clear fluid without any smell. As it dried, it felt a bit gluey – just cellular liquid.

The next day, I went to my GP, and she said I probably had an infection that caused some fluid loss. Some? By that time, I needed to change the pads in my pants every two hours. She asked me if I had forgotten to remove a tampon. I felt horrible when she asked this question. I told her there was no chance of that. Yet, she still wanted to check.

This was the first of many moments where I tried explaining something and felt that no one listened to what I said.

Since I started writing this book, I have heard so many similar stories from others with cancer or other long-term diseases and sicknesses. There is a distinct disparity between bedside manners, empathy for the patient, and just how disassociated some doctors/medical professionals can become over time. More on that later.

"Where does all this liquid come from, especially as it has no smell?" I asked her.

"You wouldn't notice it if it did," she said.

To this day, I still don't understand why she said that. It-did-not-smell. My words, descriptions, and worries were minimized to the point of being irrelevant. She did not like to be questioned. And so, this doctor's appointment felt disturbing—lots of assumptions, too much prejudice, and extremely little guidance. Though she did refer me to a gynecologist to see the same day.

Fortunately, the gynecologist gave me the feeling he was taking me seriously. All seemed to look good, and even on the ultrasound, he could not see anything wrong. He did find a tiny hole in the vaginal wall where liquid came through. He assumed this was a fistula that needed attention. It usually doesn't heal by itself.

So, two days later, I went to the hospital to have a colonoscopy to find out what was happening. The preparation for the first solved the 'bathroom issue': I could finally poop again. What a relief! Moreover, my belly ache was gone! And with it, that deep indescribable feeling.

During the colonoscopy, some cells were found that looked unusual. Then, a second colonoscopy was scheduled to look at the place again and to take a biopsy. Being admitted to the hospital, I felt too healthy to be in there, but being released after four days also felt weird. The liquid loss slowly got less and less and the medical team told me not to worry.

A couple of weeks later, I went for an MRI and a review with the surgeon to go over the results. She confirmed that the colonoscopy showed changed cells. Still, given that my belly ache was almost gone and there was less fluid, she said she did not think anything malicious was going on. It all indicated a precancerous cell change.

Just to be sure, she'd refer me to a different hospital.

I remember calling my daughter.

"Nothing to worry about. Easily treatable."

Next, I needed a proctoscopy exam. Wow! A whole new world of scientific jargon and medical procedures was opening up. I had never heard of a proctoscopy. A proctoscopy (also called rigid sigmoidoscopy) is a procedure to examine the inside of the rectum and the anus, to find hemorrhoids, tumors, polyps, or inflammation and bleeding. It is not as deep as a colonoscopy, and no anesthesia is required.

My work was quite stressful at this time. I had some struggles at work. It felt to me like I was constantly playing strategic chess and carefully considering every move I made and its future impact. My private life, however, went great. I had love in my life, someone I felt close to and at home with which gave me energy and a positive boost. I was worried and, at the same time, I was not—I think I was more annoyed that I was sent yet for another examination.

During the procedure, they retook biopsies from the area where there seemed to be a change in the cells. One of the doctors said they could feel something hard. They decided to take an extra bit from that place. For the first time, I heard it could be "AIN 3". Anal intraepithelial neoplasia. Neoplasia means abnormal growth of cells or tissues, and intraepithelial means within the layer of cells that form the surface or the lining of an organ or skin.

The three stages of AIN

AIN stages, according to cancer UK, refer to how abnormal the calls are; the cells are slightly (1), moderately (2), or severely (3) abnormal. AIN1 is called low-grade AIN. AIN2 and AIN3 are called high-grade AIN.

AIN 1: abnormal cells are in one layer of the lining. Usually harmless but can develop into AIN 2.
AIN 2: abnormal cells are in multiple layers.
AIN 3: abnormal cells are in all layers. The cells are severely abnormal but easily treatable.

At home, I started researching. Treatment would be needed because the cells have already changed so much that they're unlikely to get better by themselves. There was a risk of developing anal cancer, but the chances were exceedingly small. So, I kept being told.

The hospital called me back and corroborated the doctor's concerns. The biopsy confirmed that it was AIN3. Changed cells. Precancerous. They suggested one more procedure: a complete anal mapping. I had no idea what that meant. An anal mapping procedure is performed under anesthesia, where samples are taken from each quadrant: twelve tissue biopsies in total are taken from the anus.

On the morning of Friday, December 9, I went into the hospital for my 'anal mapping'. They told me I'd be home later that afternoon. The next memory I have is the surgeon waking me up. I remember trying to focus on him. I was still feeling the effects of being under general anesthetic. Half in the room, half somewhere else. I heard him say only three words before I fell back into a medically induced abyss: "I am worried…"

Those words echoed in my head when I left the hospital. I had to wait one week for the results. With Christmas coming closer and plans to spend it with Mom and Dad in Germany, I called the hospital numerous times to schedule an appointment for the results. The only available time they had was December 29.

Waiting was hard. On the other hand, everyone I told about it pretty much said the same thing: if it were malicious, they would call you in much faster.

On December 22nd, I am on the highway driving to Germany. It is not just me but also my daughter and her boyfriend. I love flying down the highway, and especially now, the long drive is a great distraction. The car is filled with Christmas songs and laughter.

My phone rings. It was the hospital wanting to schedule an additional MRI. I ask why. Apparently, the surgeon would like to have this for when we meet. We plan it for December 29, just before the surgeon's appointment. A worried feeling creeps in. I try and push it away.

Christmas feels surreal. I enjoy spending time with family, but at the same time, I am not there, in spirit. I just want to know what is going on. And what next? On the morning of the 29th, I have the MRI and the appointment with the surgeon. My daughter asks if she should come along. I tell her there is no need to come with me, I feel fine. She'd only be there to sit and wait for me as the MRI would take about half an hour. I expect the AIN 3 to be confirmed and then to discuss a treatment plan.

9 a.m. sharp, I walk into the surgeon's office.

9:03, I hear the words 'stage 3 anal cancer'. Not the pre-cancerous AIN stage 3?

No! Stage 3 cancer.

I lose all sense of focus. The surgeon keeps on talking. They want to give me a temporary artificial exit, a stoma, in preparation for treatment. At the beginning of next week.

Say what now?

A stoma?

Next week?

Shocked, I manage to ask him about survival statistics. He says numbers are cruel, but more on that later.

How about immunotherapy? I ask. Not because I know what it is, but because I am searching for possibilities. He states there are no immunotherapies for this type of cancer. (Don't panic, this is not the case!).

He tells me he needs to go and asks if I need a moment alone in his office.

'No, thank you.'

That is the last thing I want. He doesn't ask me if I am there by car. If they should call anyone for me. If I can leave by myself. There is no real understanding of what hearing such a diagnosis can do to a person.

Never before had I felt this overwhelmed. I didn't know what questions to ask. I was so out of my depth. It was like floating on a raft with no paddle at the complete mercy of the elements. Look out, wild waters ahead! Who was steering this ship? Not me, that's for sure! There I was—I had forgotten my life vest, holding on to the canoe's sides, flying through the rushing waters that drowned out the sound of everything else. There was nothing I could do, except hope for guidance and direction. The surgeon left. I was all by myself.

At 9:06 AM, I sent out a text message to my loved one.

"Cancer Stage 3…Fuck!!!"

I somehow left the office and for quite some time I sat on a bench in the hospital, watching people go by. Wondering how many had also just received a devastating diagnosis. My daughter didn't hear from me for two hours, probably adding to her worry. But somehow, I needed to get myself ready to tell her. It's not easy to receive the news. It's even harder to tell it to the people you love.

I still have a difficult time recalling this day. I remember her breaking down. I remember her crying. I remember myself crying. But I don't remember any of our conversations.

My calendar quickly filled up with appointments:

30 Dec   Make an appointment with a Stoma nurse.
2 Jan   A nurse will determine the exit (the replacement hole for my anus) on my belly, mark it for surgery day and show me how to use the stoma.
11 Jan   Appointment with an anesthetist for the stoma surgery.

Treatment starts six weeks later.

The 2022 New Year's celebration was supposed to be extra special this year—spending it with four cousins and their partners, their children, my daughter and her boyfriend. A happy picture-perfect family during the holidays. Having lost many dear family members over the past two years, we wanted to spend some quality time together. Here I was, hiding a one-day-old cancer diagnosis. Somehow, I succeeded.

2023 started foggy. On Monday, January 2nd, my daughter came with me to the hospital. It was one of the most surreal moments—I felt disoriented in a way, the entire situation made me feel shaken. And I am not easily shaken, but the unfolding events felt so out of control.

The stoma nurse started asking me a bunch of questions:
Are you in any pain?
—No.
Is sitting difficult?
—No.
Do you currently have problems with defecation?
—No.

Did anyone explain the details of the procedure?
—No.

The nurse looked confused. He told me he was called during his lunch break to schedule me in and didn't know what was going on. I gave him all the information I had, but while talking, I came to the conclusion that something was off. The appointment ran its course, and I was measured on the belly where the opening for the artificial exit would be cut. Yet, standing there with my shirt up and marks drawn onto my skin, I decided I would not have this surgery before I had a second opinion. The diagnosis was only a few days old. I hadn't even seen the oncologist yet. Wasn't I supposed to? I needed a pause and gathered my thoughts.

From the stoma nurse straight to the anesthetist, we encountered the second strange experience of the day. The anesthetist looked at me and asked why I was there. Why am I here? Why didn't she know? She was as confused as I was.

Leaving the hospital, my mind was made up. I did not want to stay and go through treatment there. I would still go ahead with the MRI that was planned for Wednesday. I would meet the same surgeon who gave me the diagnosis the week prior. And I was determined to get a second opinion referral to a specialized hospital. One that knew why I was there in the first place!

The days leading up to my meeting with the surgeon, I spent researching. Preparing myself not to feel so exposed, helpless, or lost as in that first appointment. At the next appointment, I would have the one thing I didn't have last time: knowledge & support.

Together with my daughter, I went to the appointment on Thursday, January 5, armed with four sheets of paper. This time, the pen would be mightier than the scalpel. I had all my questions printed out. Questions I needed answers to. As soon as we entered the room, I blurted out that I would like to be referred to a specialized hospital for a second opinion. I saw his expression change when I explained I had no trust in my treatment approach, given my experiences.

He told me it was not that easy to get a second opinion. Everyone asked to be treated in this specialized hospital, but that he'd complete the paperwork and make a referral. I told him how I felt after the anal mapping procedure, when he woke me to tell me that he was "worried." Still in the haze of anesthesia, I instantly forgot the second half of the sentence—what he was worried about. That stayed with me for quite a while: it clouded my thoughts and made me feel scared. When I finished talking, he kept quiet and just looked at me.

I then told him about my experience with the stoma nurse and anesthetist. Trying just to make sense of such a harsh diagnosis while not feeling safe or well-guided by the hospital and their protocols leaves you feeling utterly insecure, overwhelmed, and helpless.

Also, telling me there was no immunotherapy for my type of cancer—this information was just incorrect. When I asked about immunotherapy, I didn't know that it is only recommended as a secondary treatment option. He could have explained that to me. Sitting in front of him, I was prepared. I knew the name of one example of immunotherapy medication, when it was developed, and when it was first approved for usage in Europe.

It was the weirdest thing—I felt good for a moment and felt like I had won a little battle, even though I had won nothing at all. But, looking back, I think it was just the feeling of having control. Even if it was just for a short moment.

In the end, getting into another hospital for a second opinion turned out to not be a problem. The new hospital immediately laid out the process to follow. I think with anal cancer being so rare, contributing just 1%-2% of all cancers, this added to the reason they immediately took me on.

The day I was scheduled for stoma surgery in the old hospital, I had a PET scan at the new hospital instead. I had no idea that something like a PET scan existed.

> A PET scan uses a small amount of mildly radio-active glucose solution injected through a small plastic tube. Cancer cells absorb more of the solution than normal cells and will show up brighter on the scan.

If only I had known! After three biopsies plus a complete anal mapping, I learnt about this device with which cancer and possible metastases can be spotted. I definitely would have asked for that option right after the first biopsy, if the doctors needed a second test.

A week later, I had an appointment to get the results. My daughter was by my side, yet I had a queasy feeling. I remember when I saw the doctor coming out into the hallway, calling my name. I think I knew at that moment already that I would not get good news, even though I wouldn't have admitted it to myself. We entered the room, sat down and I steadied myself for what I was about to hear. The doctor started asking all kinds of questions about how I was in general. It felt like forever until she shared the results from the scan.

"It has spread to the liver, which is generally not good news."

These twelve words that flowed so easily from her mouth hit me like a ton of bricks. It was the vaguest term: "generally not good news." What does that even mean? There were so many better ways she could have shared this information. She could have looked at my file and taken into account my journey. For her, this was just another diagnosis to deliver. For me, this changed everything. Stage 4 cancer?! From pre-cancerous AIN 3 to cancer stage 3, and now this? From 'Don't worry, it's easily treatable' to 'generally not good news.'

My daughter on the chair next to me started shaking. At one point, the whole chair and floor around her seemed to be shaking.

I asked the doctor what her words meant but she didn't give a clear answer. At a certain point, I started provoking to get a clarifying statement. I asked her if I would make it through the year.

"I don't know. We will start treatment despite—"

I cut her off. Despite? Despite what?!

I asked: "Should I live out my days with the quality of life I have right now? What do you mean?"

"You would develop some 'nasty issues' if not treated. You should go home and think about things."

I couldn't even ask what 'nasty issues' she was referring to. I had no idea how much time I had, or did I have any time? How could I process this and make a plan based on information and facts? Right now, I had nothing. Just those twelve lingering mortifying words: "It has spread to the liver, which generally is not good news," of which I didn't know how they would impact my life.

We left, utterly bewildered, with more questions than answers. Drifting back into the fog.

Find a specialist
Most general hospitals rarely treat anal cancer. Make sure you have as much of a specialist as possible for your type of cancer treatment. Ask your hospital how many anal cancer cases they see every year. Many doctors have never even seen an anal cancer patient and have 0% experience with it.

Always take someone with you to your appointments
It can be so overwhelming that you forget 80% of what was discussed by the time you leave. If you don't have anyone to go with you, take a journal and capture all the information. As you go through the process, there will be many things that might not make sense or even sound contradictory. Taking detailed notes during appointments can help clarify anything that may seem unclear. The journal will help you remember and keep track. Or simply ask to record the conversation. The medical terms can be confusing. So, remember not to be rushed. Just repeat the question if something is not explained properly. They are getting well-paid, and this should be part of the package: clear and transparent communication.

You will need to do your own research
Or have someone else do it for you. Don't assume the doctors will do it for you or even with you. Become an informed patient! Only then you will be ready to ask all the necessary questions. Thinking about your diagnosis will send you on a significant medical journey. It is crucial to understand each of the steps you will need to go through, and you will need to get yourself ready for.

Get a second or even a third opinion
One of the questions I wish I had asked is how time-sensitive it is to start treatment. You may have more time to think things through and get as many opinions as you need to feel comfortable with the direction of a treatment plan. Is it a life-threatening situation or is there time to consider all the different options?

2. On becoming a cancer expert

There was this movie when I was young, an eerie John Carpenter movie from the 80s: *The Fog*. You see the mist crawling in from the sea, swallowing everything, and as you hear the boat bells ring, you know it is bad—the fog swallows and kills people. I remember how unnerving it was. Now, it felt similar. There was this fog rolling in that I couldn't see through. I didn't know how to face it. Not sure what to face, how to hide from it, or get to the other side.

My reality had shifted once again. From an easily treatable AIN to Stage 4 cancer. From a light mist to the thickest of all fogs. I couldn't believe it. I was devastated, for the way the doctor explained it, it seemed I didn't have much time left. How much time? No one could give me an answer. Back from the hospital, I sat down behind my laptop and stayed there for hours. I began digging a hole through the Internet's mountains of information for anything that would help: stats, figures, and medical research papers. Searching for anything to help me find out what to do with this *'generally bad news.'*

I asked myself, these days; in 2023, where did we stand in terms of cancer treatment? Working in Tech, I see breakthroughs regularly. It is an amazingly fast-moving world, and I hoped cancer treatment would be the same. In Tech right now, the rapid development of artificial intelligence (AI) is just revolutionizing the world and various industries. Even in healthcare, AI-powered diagnostic tools can analyze medical images with unprecedented accuracy, aiding in early detection and treatment planning. Yet, in the area of cancer treatments it seems that despite significant advancements in targeted therapies and immunotherapy, the real progress in treatment is made where pharmaceutical companies and research funding are "concentrated."

In the early 2000s, breast cancer treatment primarily relied on traditional chemotherapy and radiation therapy, with limited options for targeted therapies. At the same time, advancements in prostate cancer treatment saw the introduction of hormone therapy and targeted radiation techniques, significantly improving survival rates. This example highlights the disparity in research focus and treatment innovation across different types of cancer. Anal cancer is rare, which means that there is limited focus on it. As a result, it seems we're still mostly applying the same methods from the 70s: chemoradiation. And that's if you're lucky to live somewhere with access to basic cancer healthcare.

Aside from scrounging the Internet, I bought books. There aren't many out there, but it is good to get the perspectives of those who have dealt with cancer themselves. In the back of this book, there is a list. These books showed me the type of questions I needed to ask in order to prepare for the times ahead.

> Questions like:
> - How big is the tumor/ are the tumors?
> - Where are they precisely, and how widespread?
> - Are the lymph nodes affected?
> - What do different hospitals recommend?
> - Who specializes in what areas?
> - Are there any clinical trials I could take part in?

The medical records stated that I had a primary tumor of 3.7 cm in my anus. Moreover, there was a secondary tumor, a metastasis in the back of my liver, of 1.4 cm, and there were two spots in the front, 2 mm each. Hence, stage 4. Further on in the book is a chapter on liver metastasis with an explanation.

Since anal cancer is rare, I figured I needed a hospital that had the most experience with it. It was hard to find the right information. And there were so many other questions to be answered.

> Are you in pain? Any physical discomfort?
> Do you need pain relief?
> How was your health before the diagnosis?
> Are there any complicating factors?

The thing was, I felt fine, which was one of the hardest things to grasp. I wasn't experiencing any pain or discomfort since the initial constipation. It was hard to believe I was sick. I had stage 4 cancer with almost no symptoms. How? I did not look sick. At the time, the idea that I would have to tell people, again and again, about having cancer, actually felt sickening. I couldn't understand how my life had taken such a turn. It was suddenly not my life anymore; it was led by an illness that took over control and left me just as a participant. Suddenly, I had no right to make plans anymore; no right to dreams, wishes, and hopes. I had to push myself to focus.

> Insurance: what is and isn't covered?
> What about work? Medical leave?
> Financially, what should I expect?

All these questions and more needed to be addressed. For two days, I was glued to my laptop. Luckily, this is something I'm familiar with and something I'm very good at. I focused on treatments. First, I needed chemo-radiation to get rid of the anal cancer itself. Once that was done, it was time to tackle the liver.

Online, I found a clinic in Switzerland that specialized in liver metastases and operated on cases like mine. Armed with that information, I rang my doctor in the hospital in Amsterdam and told her about the clinic. Earlier, an MRI had been scheduled for two weeks later. I wanted one now. I wanted to act fast. Again, another bewildering dialogue occurred.

"There is a waiting list for an MRI," the doctor said.

"Well, let me buy one somewhere else in a private clinic."

She said no. I asked why. The response was that they couldn't be sure it was of the same quality. Then there would be a process to transfer the MRI results from the other hospital, so altogether it would not speed up the process. At this point, I felt like I was wasting valuable time. I told the doctor about the clinic that I found in Switzerland and that they could operate on the liver metastasis. The answer was: "There is no need for that. We can do that too."

"You can do what?"

"Operate on the metastases."

"You can?"

Since when was this an option? This was never mentioned in my last appointment.

"Well, you were not even sure if you wanted treatment."

I had never said that. That day, when I received the diagnosis, I just needed to gather myself. Collect my thoughts and process the news that I had stage 4 cancer. After the diagnosis, I was in pure shock. When I asked if I should take the quality of life I have right now and just live out my days, I tried to be provocative to get more information, a concrete outlook, a plan, guidance, and answers. Why the doctor thought I didn't want treatment is beyond me. I told her so.

Surely, many people have different experiences with their doctors. The fact remains that you might get one who behaves like mine did. One that doesn't take the time to connect with the patient. This particular doctor did not give me the feeling that I was 'the manager of my health', or that I played any role in this journey. I had the feeling she didn't want to listen to me. Instead, she just wanted to tell me what to do.

Now what? I got into this hospital for a second opinion with a new doctor. How could I trust this doctor now? This was not how my health journey was going to play out. I needed to find my voice back, I needed to find my path.

In retrospect, the medical professionals from both hospitals could and should have taken more time with my case. And yes, I understand that I am only one patient in the long list of people they treat every day, but if I hadn't been vocal during my cancer journey, I would not have received the treatment options that I eventually got. I am still so relieved the second doctor said she wanted to start chemoradiation first, and then, if necessary, ask the surgeon to make a stoma. Had I blindly followed the first medical professional's advice, I would have had an unnecessary invasive procedure and a life with a stoma.

To this day, I am happy that I asked for a second opinion and learned to be my own advocate and council of my own health and treatment plan. I had a conversation with one of my cousins. He (young, smart, successful in business, well educated) told me he would have never done what I did. Not because he couldn't, but just because he would not have seen the necessity—he would have relied on the doctors and their opinions to tell him what to do and when to do it, as they are the specialists for the situation.

Some doctors have old-fashioned ways of doing things. They are not used to being questioned. Or having to think with their patients to see if there are maybe alternative directions available. Think of it this way: when you start a contract with a gym today for a personalized schedule, in addition to the general guidance on how to use the equipment, you'd expect to receive personalized instructions from the trainer. During any course you attend, you'll judge it by the personal attention to detail and the clear instructions you get from the trainer.

Yet, when talking with doctors, we accept answers and advice that is generic rather than personalized. If you ever have to face a cancer diagnosis, remember this: no one should make choices for you or your body without consulting you. You should expect that everything is explained to the level of detail you need, and that you are made aware of possible alternatives.

I think many doctors still have a narrow vision because they are so detail-oriented in their specific field. Every cancer case needs a personal approach, but hospitals are always pressed for time. Not once but several times, I found myself before a doctor who didn't have the right information in front of them. If the right information was there, they frequently hadn't taken the time to properly read it.

To be repeatedly greeted with inaccurate information got old very quickly. It puzzled and frustrated me. It was made worse by the fact that my doctors weren't taking the time to listen to me. In my experience, communication is something that still needs much more attention in some hospitals. I recently heard the quote that medicine is the new religion. But blind faith in any situation is a risky gamble, especially so when your health is at stake. The best approach is to challenge everything until you feel comfortable.

> **Ask your doctor**
> Looking back, the most important question I would now ask after getting the diagnosis is: "How life-threatening is it at this very moment?" Many cancers are slow growing and even though the situation might look and sound incredibly scary

> at that moment, there may be no need to rush. If only I had known that I could have taken some weeks off, calming down and thinking things through. It would have helped me get more organized and put together more questions and research before treatment began. I would have had fewer surprises or things to deal with that I hadn't seen coming.
> Take time to learn about your cancer, including all treatment and care options and repercussions.

The preparations started:
26 Jan   MRI of the primary tumor in the anus.
30 Jan   CT scan of the torso to check metastases.
30 Jan   MRI and placement of tattoo dots that function as guiding points to target the irradiation field as precisely as possible during radiotherapy.
31 Jan   Meeting with the oncologist to discuss chemo treatment.

My treatment plan consisted of thirty-three rounds of chemo-radiation to get rid of the anal cancer and clean the lymph nodes of cancer cells. Starting at the beginning of February, five days a week. A kickoff with one IV drip, then continued by targeted chemo tablets in the morning and evening. Then, after this round of treatment, we would tackle the liver metastasis.

I thought there was only the standard medicine to rely on. Before I got ill, I probably would have made comments about how not to fall into the trap of questionable healers and healing methods. And rightly so. However, I learned that there is so much more out there. Natural remedies have been used for thousands of years for healing. During my research, I realized there was much more out there to consider in terms of lifestyle and nutrition. Not to replace regular medicine but to assist it. Regular medicine AND an alternative approach.

Before starting chemoradiation, I changed my dietary regimen. My sister shared articles with me on how intermittent fasting could reduce chemo-related/ induced side effects. I was so scared of the impact that chemotherapy might have on me. Yes, please, anything that could help, I thought to myself. I tried it out—I picked the easy one, wanting to be careful and not to take too much energy from my body—the *16 to 8* fasting, meaning you eat within an 8-hour time window and fast for 16 hours. In reality, this meant I just skipped one single meal, which wasn't too hard but seemed to do the trick.

I was never nauseous during chemotherapy, not even the first day when they gave me my one and only chemotherapy infusion. Every weekday, I started my day with two chemo tablets, always at the same time at 8 AM. I drank 350 ml of water one hour before my radiation treatment and then went to the hospital for radiation. Every evening at 8 pm, I again took two chemo tablets. The first week flew by, and I was anxiously waiting to see what my body would do and how it would react to the therapy.

During a video call the week before treatment, a nurse informed me about the process, like where to go for the radiation, and what kind of appointments would happen. I asked her if I would be able to drive to the appointments, or if I would need to arrange transportation. She told me I could drive there for the first week by myself but would most probably need transportation arrangements thereafter. So, I waited for nausea to start and muscle weakness to occur, expecting that I would need help.

My daughter initially wanted me to stay at her place for the weeks of treatment. Not being sure what to expect, she took her whole apartment apart, trying to make it as bacteria-free as possible and to prepare it for me being weak and needing physical support. After staying with her for only three days, I went home. We agreed that if I needed help, I would come back.

There was a moment when I asked the doctor if I should give away my dog for the duration of the treatment. She frowned at me and said that chemoradiation had no impact on animals. I did not fear that the treatment would have a direct impact on my dog and that I would irradiate him, but I wasn't sure if I could walk and take care of him. If you are no cancer treatment expert, how would you know?

In the end, I was fortunate: I could drive to all appointments and recover at home by myself. Given the quite challenging side effects that started to happen after week 4, it felt much more comfortable to be at home, just because I could walk around bottomless and not worry about anyone else in the house when struggling with the private bits.

The first week went by and I felt pretty good. Probably, because I expected the worst. I had a control appointment with the doctor to see how the treatment went and an appointment with a nutritionist to discuss my current diet. I had always been quite conscious about nutrition and had previously adjusted my food habits to manage lupus, an autoimmune disease. This is why I had a relatively carbohydrate-free diet. As carbo- hydrates and sugars promote inflammation, I left those out, which helped me manage the lupus flare-ups quite well.

The nutritionist advised me to increase my carbohydrate and protein intake by 20%. It would help minimize weight loss and give my body the extra energy it required to deal with the therapy. I told her about having lupus, yet she advised me to do it anyway. How could I increase my consumption of certain foods when I'm actively avoiding those foods *because* they aggravate my lupus symptoms? It was oxymoronic, but it was medical advice. She wanted me to eat easy-to-digest food like white bread, for example, as it would help me not get diarrhea.

I changed my diet and ate things I usually don't eat. In quantities, I wouldn't normally eat. During the weekend, my body started feeling bloated. To lift my carb intake by 20%, I started to eat potatoes, noodles, and rice. It did not take long for my joints to start hurting. I started limping in the morning to the coffee machine. In retrospect, I think what I needed was consultation, customized advice, personalized to my specific situation. It only took about a week for me to reduce the carbs again.

This was the moment when I started questioning the medical advice! I reflected on it with common sense and adjusted accordingly. I started becoming the decider of my own faith again. I researched more on what else can be done to support cancer therapy, going in all directions ranging from nutrition and mindfulness to anything that could have a positive impact.

By the end of the third week of therapy, on February 24th, I came across a book that would play a big part in my journey and still does to this day. Ann Cameron's *Curing Cancer with Carrots*. I remember thinking the book had a weird cover and an even weirder title. I mean, a carrot is a standard vegetable in the kitchen. And they're cheap. There are many so-called superfoods out there that would have made much more sense to me.

When I read that she was a children's book author, the cover made sense to me, as it had a children's book quality to it. Then I read the reviews of the book. People commented that they tried juicing carrots and that it worked for them, their mom, dad, and partner. I researched the people who gave these reviews to see if they were real people, buying real products and giving real reviews. And they were. On top of that, the author did not sell carrots, juicers, juices or even sell the book at a high price.

I bought it and sent my daughter a text message.
22:09 Can I please borrow your juicer? ;)
22:25 Please, have a look at this…
22:26 Can I pick the juicer up tomorrow?
I started juicing that Saturday.

What happened next was to become a daily ritual of juicing carrots to support my body. I drank 1.2 liters of fresh carrot juice every day. This is about 3,5- 4 kg of carrots per day. The carrot book empowered me—that's how I felt. I was liberated to some degree from the fear, as I now could contribute to my journey. And not just handle the side effects but support the healing process.

> **To consider**
> Before and during treatment, discuss natural remedies with your doctor as some might influence chemo-therapy, such as grapefruit for example.
> Now, if you think about other topics than cancer, whatever you buy (product, service, or treatment), you always ask qualifying questions to make sure you made the right choice. If it feels like a good choice, you evaluate how much it costs to consider if you can afford it. This process should be the same when considering natural remedies to aid cancer treatment: consider the costs. And, in this case, the costs in terms of health: the currency is side effects and quality of life.

The first weeks of treatment went well. I was still following the intermittent fasting ritual and drinking 1.2 liters of carrot juice every day. One hour before each radiation appointment, I had to fill my bladder with 350 ml of water to move the small and large bowels out of the field of radiation. Drinking the carrot juice meant I had a healthy liquid intake guaranteed. This juice ritual also helped me later on during treatment, when I started having pain going to the bathroom.

I wasn't sure what to expect or how I would feel after the daily radiation sessions. The sessions themselves are short, about fifteen minutes in total. The positioning on the radiation table takes the longest time. This has to be as exact as possible to avoid radiation to surrounding tissue. Laying there, the radiation machine would move around me to shoot the rays into my body from different angles. The machine wasn't loud, but the position was far from comfortable. At least, it didn't hurt. Still, though, it all felt surreal.

Entering the room putting down the pants and undies is uncomfortable. Standing in my bare butt in front of the radiation device, with two nurses in the room, was intimidating, at first. One would ask to hop onto the bed of the irradiation machine. With nothing to cover myself. They would then leave the room. However, every time I lay there, I was happy that I could count down one more session. My goal was just getting through the 33. I found it surprising that I didn't feel anything during the procedure: no cramps, no muscles seized up, no burning sensations. I would force myself to stay as still as possible and strong, thinking about what I would do after I left there. Waiting for the machine to stop, the nurses to come back into the room and me hopping off the bed, rushing to the chair to put my undies back on.

Beforehand, I expected someone to be assigned to me. Someone who would be easy to reach if I had any questions and would be there for me. However, this was not the case. I was just put into a process and dragged through the steps. It made me feel unimportant to the medical professionals. I don't want to paint a picture of every medical professional being uncaring, but how the medical staff and society generally deals with these illnesses was far from what I expected.

One of the weirdest things while going to the hospital five days per week, for seven weeks in total, was that even though I met so many people in the same predicament, everyone seemed to be in their little bubble. During all this time, there was hardly any real conversation with anyone besides the standard "Good morning". Maybe I had a different picture of how it would be just because of the movies I had seen on TV.

I am sure we have all seen a movie where someone has cancer, and they are treated with so much empathy in the hospital. Moreover, the patients exchange smiles, and words of encouragement. They talk about what is happening to them, a moment of social interaction, shared between those going through the same thing.

That was definitely not the case for me, even though I tried. Every day I dressed properly—this was part of providing myself with some kind of normality. I went for my radiation appointments, behaving like I would at any other appointment. Afterwards, I'd hop off the table with a "See you tomorrow" to the nurses. Be as quick as I could to get out of the hospital and try to have a normal day as possible.

In week 4, things started to change in the groin. The skin went red like a regular burn. Walking became more difficult because of the friction. A week later, my genitals were swollen, and the skin changed into something like parchment paper and cracked open. You can imagine how painful it was. I looked desperately for something to cover the damaged skin. A cover that wouldn't move and provide friction. Silly me, I put a Band-Aid on it, not thinking that it might remove the top skin layer when taking it off.

After this quite painful experience, I asked the hospital for help. They gave me "Engels Pluksel", as it is called in Dutch, which can be used with an ointment to cover wounds, like burn wounds, to prevent and treat infection. Made of cotton, it has one soft, textured side, which does not absorb the ointment, allowing it to do its work on the wound. I wished that someone would have told me and had given me this in advance, to be prepared.

Peeing became torture. During week 4, it felt like a bladder infection, but it was an irritation caused by the radiation. On Monday morning of week 5, I asked for painkillers for the first time. Until then, I used paracetamol only.

Multiple times before, I had asked the hospital if there were any preventative measures I could take: any creams or other remedies, anything really to prepare the delicate skin for the treatment to come. All I was given were two creams- one Flamigel, a cream for superficial burn wounds, and Fagron Derma, which is a cream to protect the skin from drying out.

One of my few breakdown moments during the treatment happened that week. During week 5, the night of March 6, I found a patient guide published by a catholic clinic in Austria. It was a neat guide, in German, of course. "Guide for prevention of vaginal problems after pelvic radiation – useful things you can do yourself". It hasn't been translated yet, but being German, it was a great read for me. I couldn't believe it. There it was: all the information I had asked for, right from the very beginning, and now I found it only so late in the process. I burst into tears. I felt once more left alone by the system.

The guide was a well-put-together four-pager, informing about the changes to expect to the vagina caused by the radiation, and how to care for the vagina. It even had little sections divided by tumors that are and that are not hormone-sensitive listing preventative measures and skin care products such as fat-based skin creams for the maintenance of the acidic environment in the vagina, moisturizing and wound healing. Each product came with a short description. There was also a section on the prevention and treatment of stenosis (narrowing) and shortening of the vagina.

I felt so frustrated. The next day, on March 7, I had this guide with me. That day, there was a review with the oncologist. When she asked me how I was, I showed her the guide from Austria. I couldn't believe it: when she looked at it, she said that in Holland they can only advise about measures that are scientifically proven and therefore no such guide can be handed out. Problems are treated when they occur: they do not focus on prevention. I was baffled. The statement that they would only recommend what was scientifically proven, felt like a weapon against me, to shut me up.

That conversation boiled over into a real argument. I told her I was losing trust in the medical personnel. Which also had an impact on my trust in the treatment. I was not being seen or listened to as a patient. I am still puzzled by how doctors (not my oncologist, in particular, but the vast majority of the doctors) are not willing or open for dialogue. Most of the time, it felt like getting marching orders. "I tell you what we are going to do. Or not going to do…"

After the treatment and especially after that conversation that day with the doctor, I felt off. In that same week, week 5, I received a prescription for oxycodone, which is morphine. When the lady in the pharmacy handed me the medication, she said that something was missing. She pointed out that oxycodone is usually prescribed with laxatives, as taking it causes constipation quite often. I was double puzzled and sad.

Meanwhile, my genitals were in a horrific state, and I slowly got desperate about what to do and how to decrease the swelling and ease the symptoms. What underwear to wear became a real issue. I could not wear my normal undies. I tried male boxers, which worked for a while. I either had to have my whole bottom wrapped like a tight package, so that nothing could move, and no friction occurred, or I was just bottomless at home.

Sitting also became an issue, even with a doughnut pillow. I called my gynecologist, who was nice and supportive, but suggested seeing a gynecologist at the hospital where I was being treated; just to have the care all under one roof, for simplification reasons. That made sense to me. He knew one there and even reached out to her for me, and she agreed to see me. Twenty minutes later, he called back, and he told me I should receive a call from the hospital shortly to schedule an appointment. That call never came.

When I went to my usual treatment the next day, I was called into the radiologist's office. She asked me why she got a call from a resident gynecologist. I explained it to her. She told me that there was nothing that the gynecologist could do for me. Honestly, I would have liked to hear that from the "specialist" for the area I had issues with. At this moment, it felt as if access to other resources was blocked.

Week 5 was not my best week. The pain got worse, so I took one of the oxycodone tablets. OMG! There was no constipation, quite the opposite. Fifteen minutes later, I experienced a major belly ache, which stayed with me for a day, and diarrhea from hell. At the hospital the next day, they told me that this could not be. I could not have diarrhea because of the morphine! Even after I pointed out that diarrhea was mentioned in the medication instruction leaflet under the rare side effects, they still told me it could not be. Right. Not my day and not my week.

I needed my voice back.

3. And then there was pain

Painkillers commonly used in cancer treatment include opioids such as morphine, oxycodone, fentanyl, and methadone. These medications help manage severe pain associated with cancer. They function by binding to opioid receptors in the brain and spinal cord and by that reduce the perception of pain. Additionally, nonsteroidal anti-inflammatory drugs (NSAIDs) like ibuprofen and acetaminophen (i.e. paracetamol) may be used for mild to moderate pain in cancer patients.

Pain is a very personal experience. People might experience similar pain levels completely different. It is important to be open about the pain you are experiencing with your doctors, and to monitor the situation carefully. Morphine, oxycodone, and fentanyl are given as tablets, but if pain levels are high and constant, they can be given on the skin as patches. A patch releases a certain amount of the medication constantly to keep the painkiller level in the blood at a certain level. This sounds great, however, one needs to be aware that these painkillers are strong! After having a patch for a while you might not be able to just stop taking it and the medication might need to be carefully tapered out of your system.

I found it extremely difficult to deal with the painkiller topic and I stretched out taking anything but paracetamol for as long as I could. Fentanyl and oxycodone get a lot of media coverage these days for their incredible addiction potential. I mean, quite a few of my music heroes died of fentanyl overdoses like Mac Miller, Tom Petty and Prince. Additionally, I did watch some very concerning documentaries on Netflix about pain medication. So, I did push it out as long as I could to take any of these strong painkillers.

One of my strategies was to ask for a light valium dose. One result of the pain was that it kept me from falling asleep at night and then, of course, waking up exhausted the next day, being even more prone to being sensitive to pain. Until week 5, I did use paracetamol and occasionally quarters of 10mg valium. When the pain got worse, I tried oxycodone, but that did not work for me. The doctor suggested fentanyl. Which scared me. This painkiller is available as patches or tablets that give longer-lasting pain relief, or as tablets that are working only shortly but very fast - meaning cutting out pain within a few minutes but only lasting for a couple of hours. The last was the option that I took home with me: 5 tablets of short but fast-acting fentanyl.

On March 14th, I wrote to the doctor:

Dear Doctor,

Update medication: after the prescription of the valium, I used one-quarter of a 10mg tablet yesterday, combined with two paracetamol. I had a full 8 hours of sleep, waking up with no pain, and the whole day was super manageable. So, this seems to be a good option for me for now.

Question on fentanyl: even though at the moment I do not consider fentanyl, as the option above works, I still have a question, in case the situation changes. Below is a photo concerning the usage of the medication. Maybe my Dutch is too poor, but how do I read this? Under the section "When should you NOT use this medication", it advises against using it in my case. Could you please comment on this?
What is the interrelationship and interplay when combining valium and fentanyl? Can I take valium, and then take fentanyl the following day, if I have a peak in pain?

Kind regards,
Leila

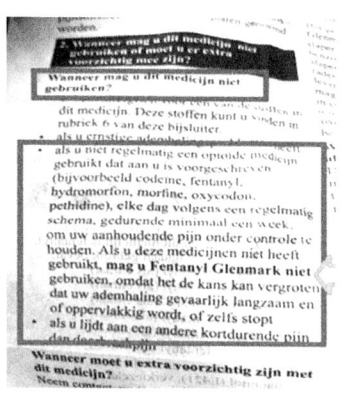

The box in the photo says: If you are not regularly taking opioid medication (e.g., codeine, fentanyl, hydromorphone, morphine, oxycodone, pethidine), every day, for at least a week to control your persistent pain, you should not take Fentanyl Glenmark (to control break-through pain) as it may increase the risk of your breathing becoming dangerously slow and/or shallow, or even stop.

The reaction I got was puzzling: they told me that the risk with fast-acting fentanyl (Fentanyl Glenmark) is that one would stop breathing, yes. However, when experiencing extreme pain, the adrenalin level would be so high that it would not likely cause you to fall asleep and stop breathing. It was up to me, they said.

Again, I felt alone. The ball (and responsibility) was given right back to me. The one who needed help and guidance. Eventually, in the last week of treatment and the week after, the pain reached a peak. I took five fentanyl tablets (not at the same time, of course). I am just happy that I didn't ask for more.

One painkiller I would like to discuss here is methadone. Methadone was given for pain management in cancer patients before fentanyl took over. It is an effective and cost-efficient option for managing cancer-related pain, particularly in patients who have not achieved adequate pain relief with other opioids or who require long-term pain management.

There might be an additional benefit of methadone for certain cancers. Scientists at the University of Ulm in Germany concluded that methadone may be able to help in the fight against cancer by making tumors more responsive to chemotherapy when administered together with the chemo medication.

> **Personal choice**
> Of course, for those who are reading this book and facing this ordeal, choosing the right painkillers is a very personal decision. It depends on various factors, including the type and severity of pain you are experiencing and what feels right for you. Make sure you are well-informed. If you are not used to these types of medications, know that your body may surprise you in how it responds to painkillers.

4. The liver metastasis
(There is hope... remember the Phoenix)

Faith whispers to the warrior: "You can't withstand the storm."
The warrior whispers back: "I am the storm."

At the very beginning of my journey, I came across this particular quote. It may have been mentioned in a survivor's success story. Some say it was attributed to Genghis Khan, but regardless of who said it first: when I read it, it resonated. I could feel a connection with it and so I had to take it on and make it my guiding quote.

When I got the diagnosis and received the words that it had spread to the liver, I automatically assumed this was the end of the line. The doctor did not say this explicitly, but her choice of words indicated there were no options left. Metastasis, the word itself seemed cruel to me. It meant my body allowed something to grow inside of me. Something I had never noticed or felt was threatening me now. It multiplied and traveled further within my body to do more damage. I felt double cheated. By myself, by my own body. Metastasis sounded to me equal to totally out of control, nothing that can be done. Something I am simply exposed to. Helplessness was something I was not used to feeling, at all.

When I started my treatment, I asked how the chemotherapy would affect my liver metastases. I learned that the type of chemo that I received was a targeted one, not systemic. This meant it would not do anything to the metastasis. It was only used to make the radiation to the primary tumor more effective. When I raised the question if it wouldn't be possible (or even better) to target the metastasis as well, I was told that the protocol is to first target the primary tumor, and then the spread.

"In this way, we give the illness the chance to show its real face," the oncologist said.

Wow.

What a tough and somehow funky statement to hear.

"But what if it spreads further?" I dared to ask.

"Then it already has, and we just don't see it yet on the scans."

As said before, I had a 1.4 cm metastasis at the end of the liver (in the back, where the so-called little tail is) and two spots in the front. I asked what those two spots were and was told that they couldn't tell as they were so small (<2mm). But the way the conversation went, it was clear to me that they expected there to be three metastases, instead of one and two benign spots. A tiny spot could already mean there were millions of cancer cells rummaging about.

Meanwhile, I was juicing carrots every day. Most of the time, I drank all the juice, 1.2 liters in one go—one glass after the other. On other days, I did half in the morning and half in the afternoon. There was no protocol I stuck to other than a minimum of 1.2 liters every day. I made further adjustments to my diet in what I would eat for lunch and dinner, plus the previously introduced eating habits like intermittent fasting.

A month later, on March 22, I had my last radiation appointment. This moment was the chance to put the impact I could have on the situation with nutrition to the test. But nutrition is no magic—it needs some time! I had barely juiced carrots for a month. In the last meeting with my oncologist, she said that we could look at addressing the liver metastases after the chemoradiation treatments were completed. When the situation in my liver was stable, without any change, they would operate. Now, she suggested waiting until September. Why September?

She explained that, by then, we would have the status review. What that meant was that if the chemoradiation wasn't successful in treating the primary tumor in the anus, they would like to perform an 'APR' surgery and remove it. So, both operations could happen at the same time, requiring only one anesthesia moment. Which is far better for the body.

APR stands for *abdominoperineal resection*. During this type of surgery, they
1. remove the anus, rectum, part of the colon, and (sometimes) lymph nodes.
2. perform a colostomy by attaching the remaining colon to a surgically made opening in your abdomen (stoma), and
3. attach a small bag to the stoma to collect stool.

The doctor told me that I was "the boss" but I should keep this option open. I asked her an interesting question: if I had this life-altering surgery would that mean that I was cured? Her answer was "no". I had done my research, and there were other secondary treatment routes that I would choose before I considered this type of surgery.

As there was no need to wait, the doctor suggested I talk to the surgeon next, to remove the liver metastases. An appointment was planned for April 20.

I knew I wanted to put natural remedies at work in the interim and was religiously juicing 1.2 – 1.5 liter of carrot juice every day.

The appointment with the surgeon was pleasant, given what it was about. It was one of the first times it felt like I was having a dialogue. I was seen not only as a case, a number, or a patient, but actually as a person with context. He welcomed me in his office in a positive way. There was even some polite humor applied. He was paying attention and adjusted the conversation to me, which made me feel comfortable. He even adjusted the conversation to the depth of information I needed.

He suggested a laparoscopic approach for removing the liver metastasis. This means only making a couple of small cuts to remove the lesions, mentioning though that there could be a slight risk of bleeding, which would then warrant open surgery. Now, I have a history of complications. At one time my inflamed appendix busted, which led to emergency surgery. The result? Scar tissue in the abdomen. Imagine a spider web of tissue in my belly. Not something a surgeon wants to reopen.

So, I raised concerns about open surgery and the possible challenges and risks. I remember he looked at me and asked me if I had ever seen the scans. I said no. No one had shown them to me.

He took the CTs and the MRIs, and together we reviewed them. My body was shown in three-dimensional slices. He patiently showed me where the metastasis resided and where the spots were. He confirmed that there would be a very small risk of bleeding, but he had to mention that this could never be completely excluded. Given that I was on my secret nutrition trial, I asked him if it would be risky at this point to wait a bit longer to perform the surgery. If we could wait just a little and let me and my body recover after the treatment journey.

I asked for four more weeks. Then, do a scan and discuss further. It was good to give myself some time, as the treatment is "not over when it is over." The radiation potency has built up so much over the treatment weeks that its impact goes on for another two weeks after the therapy has ended. In fact, the peak of the side effects is reached one to two weeks after the last radiation appointment! And it is quite a challenge.

Those are the hardest days of the whole period in my memory, as the pain was excruciating. Everybody is different, of course, and looking back, all I would like to say is: *do whatever is needed to simply get through*. Not just in terms of painkillers but, more importantly, *distraction strategies* for your days to stay motivated, push through and move the focus from the pain. After this peak, your body will slowly start to heal.

As the oncologist had previously confirmed, the surgeon said he didn't see any risk in moving out the date. We had the 'proof of time,' meaning that the situation seemed to be stable. The last CT scan was made on March 20, the new CT scan was scheduled for May 26, and the review with the surgeon for the first of June.

This was a "yippie moment" for me as this gave me control back over my life. Between the last scan and the new scan would be nine weeks. This would give me time to put this to the test, following my intuition—I felt I had to do this and that it was the absolute right thing to do.

I went on with my nutrition protocol, and a funny thing happened: somehow, I was no longer scared thinking about the next scan. Moreover, I was excited! It was not an "OMG, what will I hear next?" It was a "YES, let's do this and see what happens" situation. It put me in a much better place mentally. I also used those weeks for research on what more could be done about liver metastases and, of course, I took time to heal after the cruel treatment regimen. The weeks went by until it was time for my CT scan appointment. Finally!

June 1st came—time to see the surgeon again. My sister came with me to the hospital appointment. Another interesting moment unfolded in my journey. He said that the scans looked good but did not comment on them any further. He went on to talk about a possible date for doing the laparoscopic approach to resolve the metastases situation. Some explanation followed on how he would need to loosen the organ from the rib cage a bit, and I remember the hand movement he made. The metastasis sat at the end of the organ, which to some degree is good, but then the location was at the back of the rib cage, which made it more challenging to reach.

During my research the weeks before I came across a method called *Radiofrequency Ablation (RFA)*. A minimally invasive method using heat to destroy cells. This is done using a needle with a probe to be placed close to the tumor and then heated up to kill the cancer cells. Burn the motherfuckers down!

"How about Radio Frequency Ablation, would that be an option?" I suggested.

He looked at me in surprise, then looked at the scans.

"That… is actually a good idea!" He uttered excitedly.

Again, he looked at the scans and said that the location would be far easier to reach this way. I too was excited but also confused. Why didn't he think of it himself? The surgeon told me that if I would like to go for radiofrequency ablation, he would not be the one doing this. It was not his field. Yet, the team doing that kind of procedure was right next door and he'd just go over and ask them to join.

Then, there was the next "incredible moment" of this appointment. I asked if we could address the two spots I had in the front of the liver in the same manner.

"Oh, the spots are not visible anymore. And the metastasis is 9 mm instead of 1.4 cm."

He didn't elaborate.

I looked at my sister, and she winked at me— I felt this was the outcome of my secret nutrition project. How strong I felt!

He left the room and came back with two doctors from the other team. They looked at the scans and confirmed that the location was easy to reach for them, mentioning that it was on a perfect spot.

I asked them about bleeding risk, and they confirmed that this would be done with needles only, one with a probe placed close to the metastasis to kind of burn it away, and a second needle would be used right before, just to take a few cells that could be sent to the lab (to have information about cancer on a cellular level for possible secondary treatment). But, as there would be no cutting, the risk of bleeding would be very limited.

So, now what? He looked at me and said: You are the boss! Again, those words. And again, the responsibility to make a decision was put right back to me, the patient, not the specialist. I asked about the differences in results between surgery and RFA, and the team confirmed that the results would be comparable in my situation. Furthermore, I asked if the RFA procedure could be repeated if something was missed, or another metastasis would occur, and they confirmed that would be possible. The procedure did not erase the option of a later surgery. Therefore, I decided that RFA would be the treatment option I would go for.

Interestingly, to this day, none of the doctors have ever asked me if I did anything else to support the healing process. I mean, they must have recognized that I did quite well during the treatment, that I did not lose weight, and that my color was quite vibrant. I would expect if I were in the shoes of the doctors, I would ask out of pure interest, if there were any other measurements this person was taking.

The removal of the metastasis with RFA was scheduled for Monday, June 19th. At 7 am, I went to the hospital with my daughter and sister, and I was in an excellent mood. I would need to stay one night and go home the following day. That was the plan. Before they gave me the anesthesia, I was laughing with the nurses.

Around 8 in the morning, I was pushed into the surgery room. The procedure itself would take about 45 minutes. At 11 am, my daughter had still not heard anything. She feared something was not right. At 1 pm, she got the call from the surgeon telling her they finally managed to get me into a stable condition.

She asked him what that meant and was told that I had lost a lot of blood, which put me into a critical situation for quite a while. The operation itself had gone well with regards to removing the metastasis, but it must have hit an artery during the procedure. They could not find the origin of the bleeding and had to give me multiple blood transfusions.

My body, however, managed stop the bleeding by itself, but the doctors kept me sedated, in case they would need to perform an emergency surgery. They told my daughter they would call her as soon as there was news, and she could see me.

At 4 pm, she started panicking again. Shortly after 5 pm, the surgeon called her again to tell her that I was still in the recovery room of the intensive care unit. As soon as I was stable enough, they'd wake me up and bring me to the normal ward which would be in about an hour. One hour later, she called the hospital to ask if I had returned from intensive care to the normal ward and was told "yes". So she went to the hospital, but then on the way to the room, a nurse ran after her to tell her I was still in the intensive care unit.

6.15 pm. Every time the elevator door opened, she hoped it was me. Nobody was able to give her any information. At 7.30 pm, the surgeon called her again. She was in pieces. He told her that I was the last patient left in the IC recovery room, and they would make an exception for her to see me.

According to her, when she walked into my room in the intensive care unit, I instantly became a mum. I greeted her enthusiastically. First things mums do in these situations is tell their kids not to be worried. All my daughter saw, were all the tubes coming out of me and the bag of blood pouring into my vein. Even though I was talking to her, I wasn't fully there yet.

"I am fine, oh, my ice cream is yummy," I told her.

I fell back into a slumber. I don't remember this. Next, when I regained consciousness, I felt like I was hit by a bus. Two worried faces were looking at me, my daughter, and my sister. It was 8 pm by then. I was connected to monitors and an IV. I remember the beeping.

The nurse told me that they kept the staff for me there as they didn't know if they had to bring me back into the surgery room. I didn't know that I was kept under anesthesia for the whole day. By the end of the following day, I had had four blood transfusions. Instead of going home the next day, I stayed for the whole week.

The doctor performing the procedure was experienced but young. I could see how shook he was. He was very emphatic, telling me that he had three more patients that week and that they all went home the next day. For some reason, I got all the complications that are listed in the book and normally never happen.

Every day, he checked in with me. Weeks later, when I came for my first review, he was there to make sure everything was fine. This was quite a trip. Everything that could go wrong, kind of did go wrong. But the end result was the same. The cancer was gone!

Would I do it again and make the same decision for the same treatment?

YES, absolutely!

One thing the RFA procedure showed me is that statistics really don't mean anything. As long as you do not know on which side of the statistics you are, it is just a bunch of words. If someone tells you that you have a 90% chance to survive and you find yourself in the 10%, it sucks. If someone tells you have a 90% chance of dying and you happen to be in the 10%, it is fantastic. But as long as you don't know, it doesn't mean anything.

The risk of bleeding was minimal. When I asked what minimal meant during my last review appointment, I finally got an answer: it meant I was the second patient in the hospital to that day to whom it happened.

22 Mar	Last radiation treatment
19 Jun	Metastasis removal, Radiofrequency Ablation
08:00	Into the surgery room
	Uncontrolled bleeding
	Three blood transfusions
20:30	Back in the room on the hospital ward
20 Jun	Another blood transfusion

> *If cancer has spread and a metastasis is showing in the liver, for example, does that mean one now has two types of cancers?*
> No, if the cancer spreads like anal cancer, and a metastasis is discovered in the liver, then one does not have anal and liver cancer. The cells just traveled either via blood or lymph nodes to a different location. On a cellular level, this is still anal cancer.

5. Treatments

In principle, there are the following options when it comes to anal cancer, depending on the stage and situation:
- Chemotherapy
- Radiation
- Chemoradiation (a combination)
- Surgery
- Possible secondary treatments

I found really helpful and valuable information on the website of the Anal Cancer Foundation. Some parts might be challenging to read if you are impacted by cancer. You could have someone read it for you and give you as much detail as you are comfortable with at the moment. Keep in mind that the protocols mentioned on the website might be tailored to the US or UK, and that there could be slight differences in how things are done where you are. The overall approach, though, remains the same.

The main treatment for anal cancer is chemoradiation. This involves receiving chemotherapy and radiation simultaneously for about 5 to 7 weeks, every workday (5 days a week). The specific chemotherapy you receive may vary depending on your location. Different hospitals and countries use different chemotherapy regimens, some given intravenously and others in tablet form.

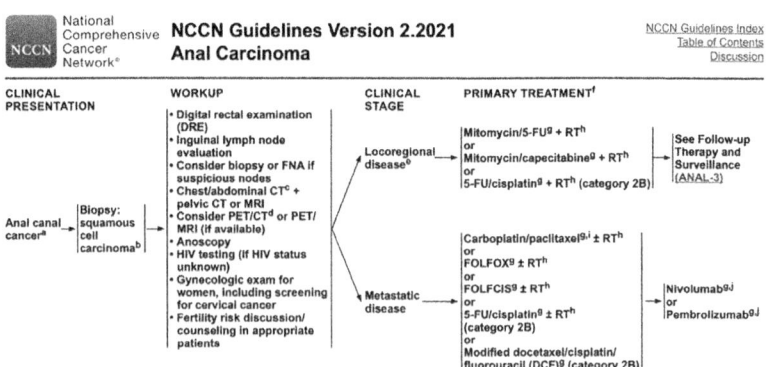

Source: www.analcancerfoundation.org/treatment/

The graphic above illustrates treatment options but remember they could vary. It is more of a general guide that you could use as a baseline to discuss with your doctor what your individual treatment path will look like. Sometimes, intravenous chemotherapy is given twice: once at the start, and again in week 5 of the treatment. For me, it was Mitomycin IV on day 1 and then targeted chemotherapy in tablet form (Capecitabine/Xeloda) every morning and every evening, 5 days per week for 33 days, plus radiation.

What is targeted chemotherapy?
As I understand it, targeted therapy means chemotherapy is given to help make the radiation therapy more effective. Chemotherapy does not automatically have an impact on cancerous cells in the body, it will only work at the targeted tumor site. Drugs/substances are used to exactly identify and attack certain types of cancer cells. Targeted therapy can be used as a "standalone", or in combination with other treatments like surgery, general chemotherapy, or radiation. For example, *capecitabine* is a targeted chemotherapy medication. It is a pro-drug, meaning a medication that turns into an active form once it enters the body.

It is then converted in the tumor, where it inhibits DNA production and slows the growth of the tumor tissue. The body breaks it down into substances that mess with the production of DNA, RNA and proteins, which then slows down the growth of cancer cells and other fast-growing cells and might cause them to die.

Targeted therapy drugs and all other drugs that treat cancer are considered chemotherapy. But important to understand is that targeted therapy drugs don't work in the same way as traditional or standard chemo drugs. They work differently in two main ways:
• Because of their targeted action, these drugs focus on the cancer cells and mostly (!) avoid normal cells. Traditional chemotherapy is cytotoxic to most cells, meaning it can damage normal, healthy cells in addition to damaging and killing cancer cells.
• Targeted drugs often work by blocking cancer cells from copying themselves (growing). This means they can help stop a cancer cell from dividing and making new cancer cells.

Radiation

Ionizing radiation kills cancer cells, mainly in solid tumors. Like surgery, radiotherapy is a local treatment. It is important to know what type of device is used, because the more precise it is, the less harm it causes to healthy cells. This is especially important with delicate tissue like in the pelvic area.

The standard type of radiation for anal cancer is delivered via *Intensity Modulated Radiation Therapy, IRMT*. There is a better device out there which is called *VMAT Volumetric Modulated Arc Therapy*. VMAT is a version of IMRT but it is technologically more advanced, basically the next generation IMRT. In addition to VMAT, it is best to also get *image guidance radiation* where daily pictures or X-ray images are made to make sure that your physical position on the irradiation bed is as precise as it can be. Every single day throughout your therapy. Having image guidance decreases the day-to-day setup variation, which allows the radiation fields to be more focused and directed.

The basis for the choice, type and lengths of treatment will be the staging of the cancer, which defines how advanced it is. There are variations of cancer staging systems, even though, generally, they are consistent. I mention this just so that you are not surprised when you see a staging that is slightly different from the one listed here.

Below is the staging system for anal cancer, based on the American Joint Committee on Cancer (AJCC)TNM system.
It comprises three key pieces of information:
- T indicates the primary tumor's size and whether it has invaded nearby organs.
- N indicates whether the cancer has spread to nearby lymph nodes.
- M indicates whether the cancer has metastasized to distant organs, such as the liver or lungs.

Additional details can be added to each category using letters or numbers after T, N, and M. Higher numbers indicate more advanced cancer.

Stage	Stage grouping	Stage description
I	T1/N0/M0	The cancer is no more than 2 cm (about 4/5 inch) across (T1). It has not spread to nearby lymph nodes (N0) or to distant parts of the body (M0).
IIA	T2/N0/M0	The cancer is more than 2 cm (about 4/5 inch) but not more than 5 cm (about 2 inches) across (T2). The cancer has not spread to nearby lymph nodes (N0) or to distant parts of the body (M0).
IIB	T1-T2/N1/M0	The cancer is no more than 5 cm (about 2 inches) across (T1 or T2) AND it has spread to lymph nodes near the rectum (N1) but not to distant parts of the body (M0).
IIIA	T3/N0/M0	The cancer is larger than 5 cm (about 2 inches) across (T3). It has not spread to nearby lymph nodes (N0) or to distant parts of the body (M0).
	OR	
	T3/N1/M0	The cancer is larger than 5 cm (about 2 inches) across (T3) AND it has spread to lymph nodes near the rectum (N1) but not to distant parts of the body (M0).
IIIB	T4/N0/M0	The cancer is any size and is growing into nearby organ(s), such as the vagina, urethra (the tube that carries urine out of the bladder), prostate gland, or bladder (T4). It has not spread to nearby lymph nodes (N0) or to distant parts of the body (M0).
IIIC	T4/N1/M0	The cancer is any size and is growing into nearby organ(s), such as the vagina, urethra (the tube that carries urine out of the bladder), prostate gland, or bladder (T4) AND it has spread to lymph nodes near the rectum (N1) but not to distant parts of the body (M0).
IV	Any T/Any N/M1	The cancer can be any size and may or may not have grown into nearby organs (any T). It may or may not have spread to nearby lymph nodes (any N). It has spread to distant organs, such as the liver or lungs (M1).

Source: www.cancer.org/cancer/types/anal-cancer/detection-diagnosis-staging/staging.html
* The following additional categories are not listed in the table above:
• **TX**: The main tumor cannot be assessed due to a lack of information.
• **T0**: No evidence of a primary tumor.
• **NX**: Regional lymph nodes cannot be assessed due to a lack of information.

The hospital will take care of the "physical" therapy, but you need to define what else you need. Keep all your options open and also consider available clinical trials. Clinical trials are studies that evaluate treatment and approaches and involve people who are currently dealing with cancer. These trials are set up to test new treatments, new drugs or maybe amended or new ways of applying existing treatments.

Depending on where you are located, there are different pages on where you can find clinical trials that are currently running or are planned to start. You can find information about running trials on the pages of the hospital that is treating you. As there are so many different sources, talk to your doctor about where to best start, but also do your own research online, as your doctor might not be aware of everything going on.

Besides chemo and radiation, there might be other treatments you might need, for example, psychological support. Your hospital most likely has psychologists or therapists they can refer you to. In my case, my employer offers a psychological crisis service, plus life coaching and reintegration services.

You do need to ask for it. If you feel overwhelmed, ask someone to ask for you! You definitely need to create strategies to wind down and find ways to relax in these confusing times. What was helpful for me were some energy therapy sessions I took, and Shiatsu once per week. Although Shiatsu is not yet mentioned consistently as a traditional form of managing cancer side effects, it is offered more and more, even directly at the hospitals.

Shiatsu treats a person's physical and mental health, which can lead to improved sleep, higher energy, and reduced nausea. If you are not familiar with Shiatsu: it is a form of Japanese bodywork therapy which is different from a regular massage and involves applying pressure to specific points of the body. It is based on the concept of energy channels or meridians through which vital energy, called "qi" flows. The word "shiatsu" actually translates to "finger pressure" in Japanese.

During the session, the practitioner uses various techniques to stimulate and balance the body's energy flow. These techniques include gentle stretches, joint rotations, and applying pressure along the meridians. For me, it was a great way to prevent side effects following cancer treatment, especially chemotherapy.

Another mechanism for me to calm down, relax and detach from stress was going to the sauna, and it still is. However, that is not possible during radiation as the skin is so fragile and sensitive, it can't deal with heat. Nevertheless, a few weeks after the conclusion of the treatment, I went back to regular sauna visits, which helped me to let go of any kind of stress and make me fill up my batteries.

Nutrition
In the very beginning when I started my research, I had a few very concerned friends and family members worrying about the same thing.

"Leila, please don't do any charlatan treatments now. Don't throw your money at questionable healers, and don't fall into the traps of alternative therapy promises".

Those remarks influenced me so much that initially I felt almost ashamed to share any findings from my research. In those early stages, I just went on the web and absorbed any information. It was difficult to immediately put the found information into a "valuable" and "not valuable" bucket. At this point, I was not objective. This is because when you are impacted by cancer, you try to look past desperation for information that can hopefully create options, possibilities, and directions for yourself.

Nutrition helped me to find my voice back, as it gave me an option to take part in my own recovery. And since my cancer journey started, I learned a lot about nutrition that I still use every day. One of the most interesting learnings for me was to understand that micro and macronutrients are not the only benefits that plants, fruits, and vegetables have to offer.

Until I started researching, it was my opinion that vitamins, minerals, and fiber protected against chronic diseases. However, recent studies show quite the opposite, as there seems to be an increase in the risk of diseases associated with large doses of random supplements. We know plants have the power to fight chronic disease, including cancer—but from the prevention point of view, it doesn't necessarily seem to be related to vitamins and minerals, but to the plant's phytochemicals.

I had never heard of phytochemicals, at the time. Plants contain thousands of phytochemicals; we don't even understand how most of these work exactly and what they could help us fight. Phytochemicals are bioactive compounds produced by plants for their protection. Most of the plants have roots and cannot run away in case of danger; they need to develop other strategies to fight predators, diseases and infections caused by microorganisms like bacteria.

In a way, these strategies are natural pesticides used by the plant to guarantee its survival. Phytochemicals have antibacterial, antifungal, and insecticidal functions that fight attackers and allow plants to survive in challenging situations and conditions. A well-known medication derived from a plant phytochemical compound is, for example, aspirin. Originally, salicylic acid was extracted from willow bark, but now it's typically made synthetically.

So, let's talk carrots
Back in the day, my dad always used to tell me to drink carrot juice. He would go and buy all these expensive organic juice bottles and when I tried to drink it, it made me nauseous. I hated the taste, but I never knew how to tell him. The moment he wasn't around, I would empty the bottles and throw them out. Now, I found out he was right! However, there is one thing my dad overlooked: to get the most out of it, the carrot needs to be juiced right before it is consumed. Bottled juice is heated and pasteurized to give it a longer shelf life, which impacts the nutrients severely.

Fresh juice has more vitamins, minerals, and enzymes compared to pasteurized juice simply because it hasn't been exposed to high heat during processing. This means the micronutrients, such as vitamin C, vitamin A, potassium, and antioxidants are preserved and can contribute to overall health and immune function. Additionally, fresh juice retains higher levels of enzyme activity. Enzymes are natural components in fruits and vegetables that help with digestion and nutrient absorption—they are important! When juices are pasteurized, it can reduce or even deactivate enzyme activity altogether.

The carrot book was well-researched and an easy read in a difficult time. The clear pragmatic way it is written, with the addition of studies and evidence in the appendix, helped me to keep my head clear while reading. It triggered me to research even more broadly, not only on medical options or the power of the carrot, but on nutrition and its connection with cancer in general. I found that it is not a matter of an either/or decision—on the contrary, medical treatment and natural substitutes go well together.

As for carrots, we don't even know yet what they can do for us and our health. According to Cameron's book, there are two chemicals that are identified and studied in fighting off cancer: falcarinol and luteolin. Searching for carrots and cancer on the Internet, you won't find much. However, if you type in luteolin and cancer, several interesting studies pop up, confirming its anticancer properties. Luteolin reactivates previously silenced cancer suppressor genes, restoring the body's ability to regulate cell division and identify and destroy abnormal cells. Sounds too good to be true, right? But there's more.

It has anti-inflammatory properties which are great not only for fighting cancer. As stated earlier: before my cancer diagnosis, I had to deal with lupus. Now, after I started juicing carrots, the lupus symptoms simply disappeared! I can eat carbs again, but I avoid excessive amounts, so it doesn't trigger flare-ups. Nowadays, I have carbs again, yet I am mindful not to consume too many in one day, especially not in combination with excess sugar.

Until I started researching, I was not aware of the role that prolonged inflammation in the body can have in creating a foundation for cancer to develop. Studies have found that luteolin can induce apoptosis (programmed cell death) in cancer cells, inhibit cell proliferation (rapid increase), and suppress the metastatic spread of cancer cells.

When it comes to falcarinol (found in carrots, parsley, celery, ginseng, fennel, and others) research and studies suggest that its powers can inhibit the growth of cancer cells in vitro (in a laboratory setting). Additionally, falcarinol has been investigated for its potential to inhibit angiogenesis (the formation of new blood vessels), which is a process crucial for tumor growth and metastasis.

Of course, I understand many factors can contribute to getting cancer and I am sharing only my personal story and view, but I strongly believe in the meantime that we can prevent cancer to a high degree by adjusting nutrition. I further believe that even when we have cancer nutrition can help to heal. Nevertheless, what you find over and over in this little book is that you need to do your own research—no one will be able to give you all the answers.

Our bodies produce around 330 billion new cells every day. If you think about this huge number, it is not surprising that some of these cells have damaged DNA that could turn into cancer. Chronic inflammation can over time also lead to DNA damage in cells, which can cause cancer. Having a well-functioning immune system, on the other hand, can help to clear those damaged cells. So, you see, having a healthy immune system is not only crucial in fighting cancer but also in preventing it from emerging in the first place.

One thing I did not realize before my journey, and which I found very surprising, is that we all have cancerous cells in our body. They are generally removed by a well-functioning immune system before they can do any harm. I always thought you either have or do not have cancer cells in your body. Given that cancer statistics indicate that in the Western World, every third person will have some form of cancer in their lives, we really should be much more educated on this topic. Prevention is something we should all be more aware of, and education should start as early as possible at school.

Now, when I tell people about juicing carrots, I get comments like "Yes, but everyone is eating carrots and vegetables, and they still get cancer." Just think about how many carrots you need to produce 1.2 liters of carrot juice. From my experience, I can tell you it is around 3,5-4 kg of carrots per day! This means that the daily intake of components like luteolin is much higher than what an average person consumes.

Another typical comment is to be careful not to eat too many carrots, as this could lead to an overdose of vitamin A. Even the editor of this book wondered about this possibility when we first discussed the story. Before the cancer, I could see myself having made a similar comment, but that was before my research. Eating carrots in excess, like I did and still do, can make the body absorb big amounts of beta-carotene, the molecule responsible for the carrot's bright orange color and a precursor of vitamin A. This can lead to excess blood carotene which can discolor the skin. And, for sure, this happened to me.

During my cancer therapy, people who had not seen me for a while commented on my great tan.

"Leila, you look great!" People would tell me.

"Well, actually…"

Someone even asked if I had been on vacation—writing this right now made me laugh out loud! But it was not a joyful laugh. As a cancer patient on medication with possible life-altering and harrowing side effects, I honestly never worried about eating too many carrots. You cannot overdose on carrots!

Synergies
When I am talking with people about juicing carrots because they contain luteolin for example, I often hear, "Oh great, does that exist as an extract, as a supplement? "It does, however, I am not sure it will do the trick if we use it as a supplement. An additional eye-opener for me was to learn about synergies. One example is curcuma, or turmeric. I did know before that curcumin is anti-inflammatory. However, if one eats curcumin and piperine (as in, regular pepper) together, the amount of curcumin absorbed increases by more than 1000 times! Which is amazing!

After I started learning about synergies, I continued to research and look in particular for sources talking about combinations of those compounds. When it comes to flavonoids, which are phytochemical compounds present in plants, I found quite some sources suggesting that when they are combined, they are more powerful and more potent in their anticancer effects.

We need to maybe start distancing ourselves from trying to look for shortcuts, such as using supplements, and wanting to have the maximum benefits with the minimum efforts. During therapy, nutrition was difficult. All the healthy things I usually like were not good for my digestion at the time. The more fiber intake I had (certain vegetables, salads, brown bread), the less I could control my bowels, which led a couple of times to challenging situations.

Anything easy to digest worked fine like white bread, toast, white rice, pasta, crackers, soups, chicken, and eggs. I still was careful, due to lupus, and indeed some carbs worked better for me than others. The healthy foods I started again after the end of the treatment, but even then, it took time to convince my intestine to be willing to deal with fiber again. Funny enough, I never had any issue with the carrot juice.

The simplest drink I liked to drink during therapy was warm water. I had my challenges drinking lots of cold drinks, but warm water was easy, and it felt moisturizing from inside out.

> Example of a daily schedule during chemoradiation:
> • Intermittent fasting, eat between 10 am – 6 pm.
> • Start the day with hot water (with or without 1 lemon squeezed into it).
> • One hour before radiation, drink 350ml water.
> • Drink 1.2 liter freshly juiced carrots (most of the time, in one go).
> • After radiation apply Deumavan or Bepanthen derma
> • Eating – during chemoradiation, vegetables and salads give diarrhea!

Mushrooms
At a certain point, I came across medical mushrooms during my research, which I hadn't been aware of before. Medical mushrooms, also known as therapeutic mushrooms, are a group of mushrooms used in traditional practices like Chinese and Japanese medicine, Ayurveda, and herbal traditions for their potential health benefits. These mushrooms contain bioactive compounds thought to have therapeutic properties.

Reishi (Ganoderma lucidum): Reishi mushrooms are famous for boosting the immune system and have been used traditionally to promote long life, lower stress, and enhance overall health. They are also thought to have potential in fighting certain types of cancer. Watch out with Reishi, it can lower blood pressure, and mine is on the low side already. When I took Reishi I had a few occasions where I was quite dizzy. Therefore, make sure you balance the dosage.

Chaga (Inonotus obliquus): Chaga mushrooms are known for their antioxidant properties and have been used to support immune function, reduce inflammation, anti-cancer properties and promote overall wellness.

Turkey Tail (Trametes versicolor): Turkey tail mushrooms have substances like polysaccharides that can aid the immune system and improve digestion. People often use them alongside cancer treatments as a supportive measure.

Cordyceps (Cordyceps sinensis): Cordyceps mushrooms are known for their energy-boosting and adaptogenic properties. They are believed to enhance stamina, improve athletic performance, and support respiratory and immune health. Like most of the medical mushrooms, they are mentioned in relation to its anticancer potential.

Lion's Mane (Hericium erinaceus): Lion's Mane mushrooms are known for their potential to enhance cognition, including memory and concentration. They are also believed to aid nerve regeneration and promote digestive health.

Maitake (Grifola frondosa): Maitake mushrooms are recognized for their immune-supporting properties, anti-cancer properties and help regulate blood sugar levels, reduce inflammation, and support cardiovascular health.

Agaricus Blazei (Agaricus subrufescens): Agaricus blazei mushrooms are known for their immune-modulating properties and may help support immune function and overall health.

Shiitake (Lentinula edodes): Shiitake mushrooms are popular culinary mushrooms with potential health benefits. They contain compounds like lentinan, which may have immune-modulating and anticancer effects.

Active Hexose Correlated Compound (AHCC): AHCC is an extract from several species of Basidiomycetes mushrooms, including shiitake (Lentinula edodes). It is known for its effects on the immune function, its antioxidant activity, its support for cancer patients as complementary therapy alongside conventional treatments, its anti-inflammatory potential, its prebiotic effects and, especially important for HPV-triggered cancers, its potential to fight viral infections. Preliminary studies have suggested that AHCC can be beneficial for combating viral infections such as influenza, hepatitis, and human papillomavirus (HPV).

Results from a small study showed the following results: four of six (66.7%) patients confirmed HPV clearance after 3–6 months of AHCC 3g. Similarly, 4 of 9 (44%) patients confirmed HR-HPV clearance after 7 months of AHCC 1g. Even though most of these studies included only a small number of participants, AHCC is used in 600+ hospitals in Japan and has been around for more than 30 years.

As with any supplement, it is essential to purchase medical mushrooms from reputable sources. If you consider taking medical mushrooms, please do some research for yourself to feel comfortable. When they were first mentioned to me, I was hesitant, but mainly because I did not know enough about the topic. When I mentioned it to my oncologist, she, as well, was not showing any encouragement.

Learning that those mushrooms have been used for a long time, not only traditionally in Asia, but also in their hospital settings, sparked my interest. Given that some of those mushrooms have been used in hospitals for over twenty years, I feel it validates their use more so than the publication of their effects in English scientific literature. Of course, this is a very private decision. I chose to incorporate them and still use them regularly now for their potential therapeutic benefits on immune function and inflammation reduction.

When it comes to food: after the treatment ended, I tried to follow the rule of eating 5-7 fresh fruits and vegetables every day. Further, I continue to consume 500ml of fresh juice every day. This is not only carrot juice; it can also be mixed with other vegetables like celery or spinach for example. Lime, for my taste, goes quite nice in combination with carrot juice. And I love starting my days with fresh lemon juice and warm water.

My supplementation scheme after chemoradiation therapy:
- AHCC 3 tablets morning/ 3 tablets evening
- 2 turkey tail morning/ 2 turkey tail evening
- 2 Lions Mane
- 2 Cordyceps
- 2 Chaga
- 2 Maitake
- Vitamin D
- Magnesium
- Ginseng & Ginkgo
- 1 Potassium
- Bio-identical Hormone – Oestrogel (via skin)
- Progesterone (via tablets)

6. Cancer, menopause and sexuality

I was 51 and blooming. You know how you feel when you have your life together? I had that. My period was not regular, but there were no significant pre-menopausal complaints. I think every woman needs some time to adjust when the "fertile" phase of femininity is coming to an end. For me, it all started early, at 11 years old. It was a very tumultuous time, with feelings all over the place.

Now, 40 years later, it felt quite similar. The thought that I would have my very last period in the coming years was a sad one, also because of everything that was related to it. With no raging hormones driving my sexual desire, for a while, I thought I might lose my sexuality altogether. But then suddenly, I got to a crossroads—I chose sexuality and intimacy. This is a very individual pathway, where either decision consciously taken is a good one.

So, I felt ready for the change about to come, and I felt liberated… and BANG!! Cancer knocked on my door. The type of cancer that had an additional impact on precisely the area I had just made peace with. If you read through the possible side effects of radiation to the pelvic area, no matter if short or long-term, it is cruel. There is no way around it. Researching this topic, I became petrified!

I read that the vagina also falls victim to *atrophy* which is the thinning, drying, and inflammation of the inner tissue as a result of the degeneration of mucosal cells. The vagina might be narrowing significantly and might not be able to expand in length anymore. Plus, urinary incontinence could happen—to me, this sounded synonymous with the complete degeneration and death of an organ. Of course, there is no telling how bad it will be for you, personally. There is no way of predicting.

When I asked the medical staff if there were any preventative measures I could take, to at least lessen the impact, the answer was clear: "Nothing."

When I asked about the likelihood that this would affect my vagina, the answer was: "Very likely."

Were there any treatments I could consider investigating after completing the treatment? "No."

The only option given was the use of dilators to stretch the vagina. A very limited option given that this would not help to address the degeneration of the organ! I remember leaving the hospital that day, completely puzzled by the answers. There was no suggestion to maybe raise this with some other specialists after treatment. There was no encouragement to look any further at all; only this significant statement, THERE IS NOTHING!

That day, I decided to translate this statement for myself into: There seems to be nothing, but let's see what I can find out. The good news is THERE ARE THINGS that can be done after, such as *Laser Therapy*. There are a few articles on the National Library of Medicine website. Not an easy read, but they all show that there are actual therapies out there. Please note that these articles are supposed to provide indications of treatment advances. These studies might have small reference groups, but the interest in funding these kinds of studies is likely not big either. So, please take them as a direction for yourself to investigate further. You'll find them in the back of the book.

Dilators

When my chemoradiation therapy ended, I asked the doctor for the dilators that they had mentioned I should use at some point after the treatment to prevent stenosis as much as possible. The answer was that they would give them to me in 6 weeks when I would come for the review as I could not use them right now anyways due to the wounds in the area.

Six weeks sounded to me like a long time. What the dilator really is for is to prevent scarring by stretching the impacted tissue. I remembered a friend from years ago, who at that time went through a sex change and for whom an artificial vagina was being built; the recommendation was to start with the dilators right away, because once scar tissue is formed, it is difficult to reverse into "normal" stretchy tissue. To a certain degree this felt to me like a comparable situation.

So, I asked for the dilators right away and for me to have them so I could use them when I was ready. I started dilating 1 week after my treatment ended. Even though my pelvic situation is not exactly like it was before, it is close enough and I do not have any reduction in quality of life.

My advice: start dilation as soon as possible!

Platelet-Rich Plasma (PRP) treatment
(also possible when one had a hormone sensitive tumor!)
I have now done this treatment five times. The treatment is painless, just a bit uncomfortable because of the area it is addressing, however my doctor is great, and she makes me feel as comfortable as possible. When I arrive at the clinic, blood is drawn and put into the centrifuge to extract the blood plasma, while I will take a seat on the gynecological chair. The actual treatment then takes about 15-20 min to inject the plasma into the vaginal wall. There is no downtime, and I can leave right after and continue my day. As for results, right after the first treatment, the bleeding during intercourse stopped. But then this is for much more; not only for sexuality, but also riding a bicycle for a longer distance, which is now possible again. I did not even think before that this could become a problem. But if you are sitting on the narrow bicycle seat for a while, there is some friction; it took about 20 minutes until I had an issue and pushed my bike back home. Furthermore, I do not fear any aftercare examinations anymore, as I know there will be no pain.

After my last appointment, I left a happy bunny, as the doctor told me that the mucosa had started to build again a little bit. When I got there the first time, the tissue was red with tiny blood vessels visible and even when only wiping carefully over it to prepare the treatment, it already started bleeding. Now after the last treatment, my tissue is back to light pinkish and not bleeding right away anymore. From my perspective, this is definitely a great treatment that has a positive impact on my quality of life. Keep in mind: health insurance might not cover these treatments—yet. Then again, it is always worth asking. If we don't ask, it won't make it into the health insurance treatment catalogs.

And now that I have done a few treatments, I will send the reimbursement requests to my health insurance, so that they have a record of the requests.

Hopping back for a moment to the prevention of side effects, there are some things that should be considered.

Radiotherapy, without a doubt, is an attack on the body. It is impossible to prevent damage to healthy cells during the therapy—cell damage is the nature of the treatment, with the main target getting rid of and damaging cancer cells. Unfortunately, it will damage healthy cells too, it will create wounds that won't heal for the duration of the treatment, and it will cause pain.

There are quite a few creams that can help throughout the process; their use will slightly ease the acute symptoms. To give an example, the cream Duvaderm and Bebanthen have helped me to be able to go to the toilet. Both are very simple creams that have no scent. Applying a thick layer every time after going to the toilet and every time right before going again, helped to protect the damaged and open skin at least a little from getting in touch with urine, which made me feel completely on fire.

What needs to be avoided under all circumstances is not eating and drinking enough. When going through therapy, getting radiation and chemo, it is so important to eat and maintain the strength to go through treatment, as well as to keep drinking enough to flush out the poisons. But when every toilet run means utter pain, one might start to eat and drink less to avoid going too often. Strategies need to be created to not fall into this trap.

You will find a list of creams that helped me in the appendix.

It is important, though, to always keep in mind that everybody is different. Just because there is a list of excruciating side effects doesn't mean one will get them all. Furthermore, just because there are awful stories out there going through the therapy, that doesn't mean it will be the same "horrible" experience for everyone. It won't be a walk in the park, but it's possible to get through. It takes time.

Hormone Replacement Therapy (HRT)
A few words on HRT, which is a difficult topic. And I probably would have said slightly different things before and now after the cancer just because I did not really deal with the topic properly before; and did not read up on it as much, but still might have articulated a superficial statement based on a common opinion and what I "had heard" before.

No matter what, the hormone discussion is a sensitive one and again a very, very personal decision. A decision as well that only can be made if the cancer is not hormone sensitive. If the cancer is hormone sensitive like, for example, breast or prostate cancer, HRT is usually avoided due to its risk to stimulate cancer growth.

If the cancer is non-hormone sensitive however, HRT can reduce treatment side effects and ease menopausal symptoms caused by treatments like radiation, chemotherapy, or surgery. For me, the symptoms were mainly hot flashes, not being able to fall asleep or stay asleep, and brain fog. But the list of symptoms is much longer and can even include depression, mood swings, skin irritation, decreasing bone density and more. Providing an estrogen-progestin combination definitely reduced the symptoms for me and improved the quality of life.

In order to start getting deeper into the topic, one needs to understand where the "bitter taste" comes from when we hear the words *Hormone Replacement Therapy*. In the 1960s and 1970s, there was a book called "Feminine Forever" which suggested that menopause was caused by a lack of hormones, leading to issues like painful intercourse and a perceived loss of attractiveness, beauty, and youth. This was just at the time when women's roles changed dramatically, the moment of the rise of feminism.

During this time, new worlds of possibilities were created for women. It was the emancipation movement, women beginning to get equal chances in education, empowerment and job possibilities. Some of the goals of the feminist movement seem incredibly common sense for us today, and so very simple, like letting women have freedom, equal opportunities, and control over their lives. This included control of their body like availability of birth control, right to abortion and right to their own sexuality.

Which then in a way became a driver for hormone therapy (HT), which became increasingly prescribed, amazingly reaching over 50 million prescriptions annually in the US by the 1970s. However, in 1975, studies showed that using estrogen alone increased the risk of endometrial (uterus) cancer, leading to a decline in HT use. By the early 1980s, it was understood that adding a progestin to estrogen therapy could reduce this risk, which led to the development of a combination therapy and another hype in HT prescriptions.

Throughout the following two decades, there was a significant increase in HT use, supported by observational studies suggesting benefits for cardiovascular health, notably in the Nurses' Health Study. By the late 1990s, HT prescriptions peaked at an amazing 90 million annually, serving around 15 million women.

But then there was the big drop, a change once again in 2002, when administrators of a study known as the Women's Health Initiative (WHI) stopped their research. They announced that while HRT has benefits, those would be outweighed by the risks. At the time there was a study that specifically linked HRT to an increased risk of blood clots, stroke, and breast cancer.

Decades later, that study is now seen as flawed. And while the history of HRT continues to spark debates, it is evident that utilizing estrogen and progestin to manage postmenopausal symptoms is beneficial for women's health. And "health" means more than just hot flushes; it also means dementia, osteoporosis, urinary incontinence, vascular calcification, and such.

The poorly conducted trial caused a sudden drop in HRT use, leaving many women without effective treatment, despite unclear evidence of harm. Recent studies have reaffirmed the benefits of HRT for symptomatic women who are within 10 years of menopause or under 60 years old. Those 10 years are the "golden window" of opportunity to start with HRT. The window opens within the perimenopause and closes latest 10 years after the last period. During the 2002 study, the average age of the participating women was 63.2.

After the window has closed, one should no longer start with HRT, because of increased risk of thrombosis, a heart attack or stroke, which is basically due to age-related damage to vessels. It's best to start HRT when you're physically healthy. This is also the reason why the golden window can already close earlier, like within six years, for example, if one has already developed typical age-related illnesses.

Additionally, the actual medication that we get today in HRT is not the same as what was given before. In a review of past and current studies, it is painfully apparent again that a general lack of consensus still persists among providers regarding the benefits vs risks of HRT, and that is "STILL" largely in part due to the WHI study of 2002.

I think what strikes me again after my journey as so apparent is 'here we are again', with quite a big question, quite a big problem, and alone in the middle of a discussion of doctors who cannot find a consensus; again "we are the boss", needing to make the decision alone for ourselves without the guidance we actually should receive.

A couple of things, however, to clarify and mention: I made the decision to take HRT and decided on bioidentical hormones. A few times I got the comment that those hormones seem not to be "biological". And yes, they are not! They are not organic—they are synthetically produced. What bioidentical means is that our body is identifying those hormones as their own; it cannot spot the difference with the own hormones it produces.

Please do not see this section as an advertisement for HRT, but hopefully as a trigger to consider and to research on your own. While the impact of menopause can be quite significant, HRT should not be dismissed just for the wrong reasons.

Recently, I have learned that DNA based testing is becoming more available, which promises to give us a greater understanding of how our body responds to and metabolizes certain nutrients through DNA. This would help us to understand and manage (pre) menopause issues better, no matter if it is feeling stressed out, unable to sleep, sweating, dryness or struggling with anxiety.

Those DNA tests analyze estrogens, progesterone, cortisol, and other key hormone levels, and then provide a personalized nutrition and supplement program. They provide information on how our individual bodies absorb hormones; they determine the current ratio between progesteron and estrogen, and how to keep an "ideal" and most-healthy level. This is definitely something I will keep an eye out for and will consider doing as soon as it is available to me.

7. Cancer and work

The "C" word is not talked about, at least not in my environment. Slowly though, I came to an age where sometimes I found myself in the following conversations: "Did you hear so and so's spouse got cancer," or hearing that someone has not made it and passed away. Usually, it is only briefly talked about, and the assumed health status of that person is shared and that's it. More like sharing a "sensation" story.

I work in the Tech sector, which is fast paced. Goals, structure, strategies, visions, and departments are reinvented every year. One must be strong, agile, dynamic and … invincible, and forever young, while the rest is changing continuously. And I fit right in. I always referred to myself as a superhero, 3 meter tall and bulletproof (and I still do, but maybe for other reasons), clocking uncountable hours at the craziest times, accommodating multiple time zones, often saying "yes" to projects before I even knew all the details.

Once I understood the full extent, I recognized that it was about trying to make the impossible work with the limited resources I had. Then again, in my environment, we judge people by their "can do" attitude and finding solutions instead of raising issues. And I still made it work somehow. 24 hours in a day? I felt that sometimes I should hand in somewhere the request to extend the length of days by 10 hours or so. The Tech business is fast and hard—super fast compared to how some other industries conduct business.

In 2022, I was promoted to Director, which was a big deal for me. We still have so few women in leadership. First, I was promoted to regional, then to global director. However, I was still an individual contributor and without a team. I got the responsibility but was constantly challenged with the bandwidth to deliver it all. I'd deal with multiple projects, multiple time zones and quite a share of politics. The stress level went through the roof.

In previous years, I worked much more beyond my direct responsibilities, just to show I could do it and that I was ready for the next level. When I got promoted, that did not end. This came to an abrupt end when I got my diagnosis. I called in sick on December 29th when I was told about stage 3 cancer. Around the same time, my boss told me she was leaving the company. There had already been some changes: her direct boss had just left shortly before, and even though I had to concentrate on myself and my journey, I was worried about what was going to happen at work.

Two levels above me changed, while I was on sick leave; two new levels above me not knowing anything about my contributions, what I can do, the quality of my work. And often if new leaders come in, they bring their own teams with them. I was worried that I might lose my job as a consequence. There seemed to be two battles going on at the same time, that I would need to fight simultaneously. I felt so out of control. My whole life was in disorder.

Late January, when my new boss started, I received the stage 4 diagnosis. I was faced with some additional new challenges. Now what do you do? Stay away from the new boss completely while being off sick? I did have regular check-ins with our Human Resources department to discuss the status and progress of my health. And I had regular appointments with the company doctor, which might not be common in other countries, but is very common in The Netherlands, when people are out on long-term sick leave.

A company doctor is not employed by the company, but by a different entity. One of their functions is to accompany the employee during long-term sick leave and make sure they are on track to return to work as quickly as possible. They are a key component of the reintegration process.

Now, a difficult decision needed to be made. Will I reach out to my new boss at all? Will I send him an email or request a 1:1 meeting? But then what will we have to talk about? At this point, it cannot be about reintegration, I can't come back to work not knowing what the future holds. Should I talk openly about my health situation? And how do I introduce myself then?

Hello, I am Leila, your team member who is out for an unknown amount of time? (.... your team member that you cannot count on; that's how I felt weirdly enough).

Should I explain exactly what I have? Should I mention the C word, and if I would mention the C word, should I mention the type? Should I mention the word 'anal'?

Hello, I am Leila, your team member that you cannot count on, who is out for an unknown amount of time and has anal cancer?

Would this make me stronger or weaker in my position at work? What would he think of me? Would he draw conclusions about me? What would he think about how I live my life?

A cancer that starts with a word afflicted with shame. A cancer that can be triggered through HPV. Would it make me safer if I'd tell him about the HPV stats and that more than 80% of all people are infected at some point with HPV in their life? Would he ask anything or just judge? How many details should I give proactively? How would I feel if any of my colleagues or people in my organization would know? Do I want to generally talk openly about cancer, about my cancer?

My head was racing. I read somewhere that many people feel so ashamed that they refer to their anal cancer as colon cancer or colorectal cancer, just to avoid the word 'anal'. As if the word was a dirty word. It was disturbing to learn that many people hide their illness altogether from work. Pretend everything is normal and just work, work, work… While at the same time, they are battling for their life.

I remember I had a colleague some years back, whose wife, I heard, had cancer. I saw him walking across the floor every once and a while; one could see in his whole expression he was going through a rough time. From a certain point on, I did not see him anymore at the office. Next, I heard his wife had passed away. I wanted to write something to him, condolences, express my sympathies or anything but felt frozen, overwhelmed, and thought I did not have the right words. When he was back at the office, I had the feeling he was keeping his distance generally from people. I still wanted to say something, but felt unsure if I should, or how I could now?

One day, on the way to leaving the office and taking the elevator downstairs to the parking lot, he hopped into the elevator. There was this awkward silence up to the point where I spurted out my condolences. How sorry I felt that his wife had passed. He genuinely thanked me for it. I told him that I was so sorry for only talking to him now, but I didn't want to invade his space and wasn't sure if it was okay to approach him about this sensitive matter. And honestly, I didn't know how to approach him.

He told me something that made quite an impact on me: he said he may come across as though he doesn't want to talk to anyone, just because of being overwhelmed with grieving and sadness. But every message he gets—every time someone approaches him—makes him feel a bit better, helps and encourages him to take a tiny step forward. Every contact is better than no contact, he confessed. And if it is too much at the moment, I would sense it. After this conversation. I always sent a message or went to talk to people when I heard they lost someone.

So, now I decided I would talk about it openly. Not only with my boss, but generally. And the most amazing thing happened, it liberated me. Talking about it. The more I did it, the easier it got. I picked a few colleagues that I had a good relationship with and trusted, and I told them. In the beginning, these conversations were full of actual tears, or tears that needed to be swallowed down, with a shaky voice, which made me vulnerable. But the reactions were amazingly supportive!

When you talk about it, you learn how many people deal with cancer themselves. Who had it or had/have a dear friend or family member who has it. And even the ones that could not be supportive, were supportive! One, for example, reached out to wish me all the very best, but then said that he wanted to keep cancer as far away from him as possible and could no further talk about it. And we never did, but still I felt the support. Talking about it made me not weaker: it made me feel stronger!

And I scheduled a virtual 1:1 meeting with my new boss and told him I had anal cancer! He was so supportive! He allowed me to make adjustments freely. From then on, we had regular virtual 30-minute check-in meetings. Even though I was officially off sick 100%, I wanted to continue to do some work, nothing with harsh timelines or time pressure though. It felt like preparing for when I was back. Even though I felt supported by my employer, I understand that this might not be the same for everyone.

Looking back, I wish someone would have helped to form a few questions towards this topic of discussing cancer at work to make the situation a bit easier to start with. I believe that for the employers, the HR team, the manager this might as well be a situation out of the ordinary, something they usually don't see and are not as well prepared for as we would wish.

There were a few distinct feelings I went through with regards to work:

- Feeling angry and annoyed at myself, that I could not work the way I would usually do.
- Feeling worried about how people would react, how they would feel about me.
- Feeling guilty that I couldn't perform as usual, that others might need to take on some or all of my work for the time being.
- Feeling like a burden.
- And then, at some point, worried about finances.

> *My advice*
> Talk with your employer about making changes to your workplace that may even allow you to keep on working or help prepare for your return to work.

I believe not all companies will have the same flexibility, and it might depend on the size of the company you are working for and the supporting resources they have. But think about what would help you feel right in your current situation? What is the adjustment that you would need?

Have this conversation with your employer, and if you feel uncomfortable having this conversation by yourself, take someone with you that can support you and maybe even speak for you. That is absolutely okay! Only after I had been back at work, I came across a fantastic neat guide helping to formulate critical questions to ask when in the situation, covering almost every angle: *Work and cancer* (tinyurl.com/3ch8ebct).

It is mainly focused on a UK audience, but most of the questions the guide raises are applicable anywhere. One of the challenges, for example, I was not prepared for, didn't even think about at that moment, was how cancer could affect my financial stability. I knew in my case that my salary would be safe for six months and then it would drop by a certain percentage.

Looking back, I wish I had had more information available and be better prepared as to knowing what to expect. I had no idea what Statutory Sick Pay I might be receiving after those six months? How long would I get paid altogether? If being off work for a long time could affect any insurance, the pension scheme or other benefit payments?

As for counseling
How about counseling, access to an employee assistance program (EAP) and certain supporting therapy offers? Ask your employer what policies they have for your situation and where you can find this information. And if you cannot go back to work, what "health-related retirement" options are there, and who can help with that?

8. In full remission, now what?

What does life look like now? Après cancer? Well, not much has changed, to be honest. What did change is the sequence of my values. Working is still important to me but friends, family & undisturbed quality time have become much more important in my life. By "undisturbed" I mean, to be in the moment. For example, at family gatherings, I would still be keeping a close watch on my phone making sure not to miss any email. It was the same while walking the dog or doing other things. Answering emails on vacation days, and all.

Those things do not happen to me anymore…well, a lot less. During the weekend, I am off the clock. When I am out for dinner, I do not check the phone frequently anymore. I now honor quality time and am much more sensitive to what is worth spending my time on. However, I am still in the process of finding my new normal. It is a process—living life, evaluating, and adjusting. Is it worth and appropriate to work twelve hours a day? Is it okay sometimes, if yes—when? What is the right balance?

It is funny seeing me write now the word "balance". I have used this word so often. Before having cancer, the word had meaning in my life. Looking at the word now, I don't think I ever really understood what it meant. Maybe I still don't know what it means, but I am on the journey to find out. I continue to eat healthy, and even though sometimes I struggle with that, I will continue. I know how much impact nutrition can have as part of the right balance. Finding time for sport and a bit of silence still needs to happen, not just squeezed into the day but really having and setting time aside for it. I am still working on that.

Another part of the journey is to gain trust again, trust in myself and trust in my body. Am I allowed to have and make future plans again? How long out am I allowed to make plans? What is the time window? Only thinking a few months ahead? What is summer vacation going to be? Should I go hiking in winter in the snow? Or do I dare to allow myself to think more than twelve months ahead… what would I like to do next year?

An illness like cancer turns a whole life upside down from one second to the other. What was true just now, then suddenly is true no more. What was possible just now, might not be possible the next moment. It takes time to win the trust in oneself back.

Every three months, I must go to the hospital for reviews. It was amazing to learn that cancer is so rare that there is no official review protocol for it, so we had to make one. These review appointments are nerve-racking. But this is due to the issue mentioned before. The trust between me and myself has been shaken, both physically and emotionally. There is not much advice I can give on how to get through this review cycle. I can tell how I do it, though.

I try to be "neutral." Not to be positive because I could be disappointed but not negative either. It makes no sense to worry about something that might never come true. In the meantime, I am trying to take on an "ok, what's next" attitude which works for me for all scenarios.

When I went for my last review, for example, I had a CT to check the liver. All still gone, nothing else there. I then had a digital exam, and the doctor could feel a little spot inside of my anus. BUMMER! I was disappointed (with myself and the result). I asked if this could be scar tissue. The doctor confirmed that this could be the case. So, I tried not to freak out and adapted to the kind of "OK, what's next?" attitude. Next was to do an MRI and a mini colonoscopy.

I did not want any calming medication for the procedure, as I find it bearable, not painful. I wanted to be able to see whatever it was on the monitor. Follow the doctor and ask questions. And I did – and she said exactly those words – that she thinks it is some scar tissue forming. The MRI indicated the same thing, and remission was confirmed. Still, nerve-racking. But it does subside quickly. And onwards.

One other challenge with remission is that it just happens suddenly. I know this sounds weird! But there you are - you were hit with the most horrendous news, you faced it, dealt with it and then you are finished with treatment, and you are in remission. YAY! Now what? You do not get a guide or action plan to stay well. The medical and healthcare system does not provide security for this uncertainty gap.

For me, my nutrition protocols fill this gap to some degree, as I continue to participate in my healing. I try to cut out the negatives and let in more of the positives. I am certainly a more leveled person than I was before cancer. For females, there might be another challenge after rounds and rounds of radiotherapy to the pelvic area. It can send them into menopause at lightspeed. A woman might be peri- menopausal in one month and postmenopausal just the following month, which feels like being hit by a bus.

You might have night sweats where you have the feeling you are waking up in a swimming pool instead of your bed. But it can have a tumultuous impact emotionally, as well. Watch out for signs of depression! And if you are feeling low, talk about it and seek out help. Hormonal change can have a huge impact. What stayed with me were first some short-term and later some long-term side effects. Which impacts different parts of me, and I need to learn to live with them.

There are some minor things that still bother me, but hopefully they will be resolved. During the radiation treatment, I suddenly recognized that I am more stiff than before. For the majority of my life, I did Pilates, often multiple times per week. Suddenly, I find myself having issues sitting cross-legged. And my hands had difficulty reaching the floor.

I asked the doctor about it, and she said that she didn't think that this was caused by radiation. Then again, while researching, I found quite many people talking about the same issues, after they had pelvic radiation. And it makes sense: radiation impacts healthy cells, and the bands around the pelvis are definitely in the radiation field. Another side effect is that it seems harder to concentrate on things and to hold presentations. I am losing words more often and need to prepare much more than before.

I remember sharing this with someone who said then to me: "Leila, don't worry. If you start speaking and you make it beyond the first slide, you have your story, and the words will come." But this is not stage fright. If I don't prepare, even with topics that I am very familiar with, the words just don't come to mind. This doesn't mean I am not as good at my job as I was before, but what it means is that I need to be aware and prepare accordingly. It also means that I need to make my environment aware that things have changed slightly, and that I now have more challenges dealing with ambiguity.

There are other things: the skin in my pelvic area is just more fragile than before. I need to watch what I am eating, because it might impact the skin of the anus. The weirdest thing! Eating too many nuts over a couple of days might cause little hair thin cuts in the anus which hurt for a couple of days. There are a lot of little things to accept and find ways to deal with. This all has an impact as well on your sexuality.

Speaking of sexuality: Western society is weird sometimes. You would think that talking about it is no longer taboo. Additionally, if you listen to some hip hop and rap songs, they are very explicit. Then again, imagine you are in a vulnerable spot, in combination with illness. You need to address this sense of sexuality in the context of being afraid of losing it altogether, because of the impact a therapy might have. Having these kinds of conversations feels like tapping into taboo territory again. At least, I felt like that, and I am not a shy person.

It felt weird sitting in front of the doctor, hesitantly asking questions and slowly realizing the extent of impact the treatment might have on this specific area of my life. My sex life. And then trying to assess the ground I was standing on. Trying to ask and understand: but what does that mean for my sexuality? I had the feeling that for them, this was not important. It didn't matter. Getting me through this alive was the measure of success. I remember using an example for the doctor I was talking to. I said: "Well, I do not want to survive… I want to live, and that means to have a life afterwards with a certain life quality."

It was such a scary feeling, realizing that this illness might take away my sexuality altogether, something that belongs to your life no matter how much importance you give to it - it is still a part of everyone. Think of all those young people who might go through the same, young women and young men who have not even created a family yet. This is an important topic to openly talk about! Or think about single people who would want to find a partner after cancer!

I saw some quite concerning stats: after anal cancer therapy, 78% of people have a sexual dysfunction. And then, one third of that 78% gave it up altogether, and do not engage in sexuality anymore. This might not feel important to you, at the moment, as your mind might be occupied dealing and coming to terms with the current situation. But still, this is something you should address right at the beginning with your doctors and not let go because after you have been through all the procedures, it definitely wins back importance, and you want to make sure that you still have options.

9. HPV

The majority of anal cancers seem to be caused by the high-risk HPV virus, which is in 90%+ cases, in particular, strains 16 and 18. But just because you are diagnosed with it and have it, doesn't mean you will develop cancer. I have not found any source that gives guidance under which circumstances HPV develops into cancer, for sure. And some things can be done today for prevention. A vaccine is available for older kids and young adults to protect against several strains of HPV, seemingly including the ones that could cause cancer. Preferably, the vaccine should be administered before sexual activity. There are sources that say that one can have the vaccine until 45—so go and check, as it is always worth asking.

Here is the hard truth: yes, HPV is an STD (Sexually Transmitted Disease), but nearly 90% of adults between 18 and 65 have at least one train of HPV—and, no, you don't need to have anal sex to get it. You do not need to have had any prior intercourse at all and you can still be HPV positive. HPV spreads from skin-to-skin contact—yes, read that again! Skin-to-skin contact. That is the reason why condoms don't do the trick either.

Important to understand is, everybody can and will probably have it at some time in their lives. But don't panic; even if you have it, and even if it is HPV 16 or 18, this doesn't mean it will develop into anal cancer, uterine cancer, or throat cancer (due to cunnilingus). Most people won't even notice, as nothing happens. The immune system gets rid of the virus eventually, which means that our immune system usually clears out the virus naturally within two (!) years. Important to understand is that the virus can lay dormant in the body for years, decades even, without any symptoms.

If you are HPV positive, consider taking medical mushrooms, AHCC. It is an extract from the shiitake mushroom which can help your body to clear out stubborn HPV infections. AHCC is not that common in Europe yet. Doctors do not proactively suggest it, because they do not know that it exists. Though, in Japan AHCC is given in hospitals to patients for 20+ years to boost and strengthen their immune system to get rid of HPV and even herpes. I made it my daily routine to take AHCC supplements.

> *Check*
> Having more sexual partners increases the chances, obviously, or if the HPV virus infection becomes chronic and stretches over years. But this only means to be aware, go and get tested. If you have it, make sure that you are regularly checked for not only uterine cancer (via PAP tests) but also for anal cancer. It is an easy procedure, a simple digital exam.
> Checking for anal cancer is not part of a doctor's standard protocol, probably because it is super rare. You need to ask for it. Additionally, when the doctor comes back and tells you that you have hemorrhoids, just ask again to double-check because anal cancer can easily be mixed up with hemorrhoids as symptoms might be similar.

> *Had I known*
> If I think about pieces of information I would have liked to know before embarking on my journey, then one would be knowledge about biopsies. Biopsies are good to provide information about cancer on a cell basis. They will tell you exactly what kind of cancer it is and how fast it is growing.

Lately, there are more sources, medical sources mentioning taking a piece and cutting into a lesion could allow the cancer to spread. If I think about my story, I had three+ biopsies, and looking back, I am not sure if I should have allowed multiple biopsies being taken during the colonoscopies, while in retrospect anal cancer was already suspected. Today, I would not just say yes and rather discuss other options of examination, like anusycopy/sigmoidscopy and if then still diagnostic measures would be necessary go and get a PET scan.

10. Cancer and family/friends

As if you don't have enough on your plate, you will also need to deal with your family and friends' pain caused by your diagnosis. You will encounter many different responses to you. You might need their help to get you through this process. Some people react completely differently than what you expect, some people you may even lose during the whole ordeal. But you may find allies where you didn't expect them, and some existing connections will even become stronger.

Just after I was diagnosed, I contacted a friend who also had cancer. Speaking with someone who knew more about the situation than me at the time helped me a lot. He gave (and still gives) me feedback in a way that felt (and feels) right: no pity, straightforward, with humor and not feeding fear.

One of the things he said in the very beginning was to always feel what I feel without guilt. If I am feeling good, just to feel good and be happy and be my normal silly self—without guilt. If I am feeling bad, just to feel bad, and again without guilt. I didn't understand that comment in the beginning of the journey, but later on I did.

People have perceptions and opinions about how someone is and behaves with cancer, how they must be treated, and to be careful around them, how they feel, even how they look. In reality, perception and opinion don't go together, sometimes.

It helped me to dress up when I went for radiation. I wore dresses, skirts, jeans, and shirts. Some days, I even put some makeup on. I just wanted to look normal which helped to feel normal (or as normal as it is possible in this situation). I laughed and joked a lot, with the nurses when in the room being positioned for the radiation. To be in the best possible mood helped me through the days.

I had to think about the people I would confide in. I told my partner, my daughter, one of my cousins I am close with, and some friends. But certain people I could not tell. My mom was one of them. And I couldn't tell them, because I knew that they might take it hard, and I wasn't able to face this and give them consolation. I needed to be strong for myself. I could not take care of them and deal with their fears boiling up, deal with their pain and tears.

Eventually, I asked my cousin to please call my mom and break the news to her! You see, for a long time, I could not talk to my mom, because I knew how scared she was for me, and how this would multiply my own fears. Telling some people personally and not others does not mean you prefer one person over another or love them any less. It does not mean you are closer to one over the other. You need to use your strengths wisely—for yourself (which is not selfish, either).

> *Advice*
> When you are diagnosed with an illness like this, you must break free from certain norms and let go of caring about the perception and opinions that others might have of you. You have one job to do: be there for yourself and be strong to get through what is ahead of you. Get help for what you need help with to get done and do not feel guilty!

11. The future?

I believe (and hope) that the future of healthcare will be characterized by increasingly personalized treatments. As we witness, at the moment, rapid advancements in technologies such as genomics, artificial intelligence, and wearable devices, healthcare will hopefully become more tailored to the specific needs of each individual, customized to a person's unique genetic makeup, lifestyle, and environmental factors.

Today, genomic testing allows for the analysis of diagnostic information for individuals, analyzing information of disease risk, early detection of illnesses, how their body absorbs nutrients and by that identifying the most effective ways to promote health. Genomic medicine holds immense promise in revolutionizing healthcare, particularly for individuals with rare diseases or cancer. I think it will offer the potential for prompt and accurate diagnoses as well as personalized treatments that will be adjusted to each patient's specific needs. Personalized healthcare might result in more effective treatments, fewer side effects, and improved overall health outcomes for patients.

At the same time, I believe it will empower individuals to play a more active role in managing their own health. While personalized healthcare will focus probably mostly on applying standard medicine, at the same time, we will have access to much more detailed information about ourselves. Understanding more about how our body functions, how it is fueled, how it absorbs nutrients, how this changes in moments of stress, how our individual hormonal levels shift in certain situations or influence one another.

This will help us to have our own holistic view on our health and determine actions we want and need to do to improve it. Understanding the power of nutrition will play an even bigger role then to keep us healthy, because we will be able to use it in a targeted way for our benefit.

Let food be thy medicine and medicine be thy food.
Hippocrates

Acknowledgements

Thank you for taking the time to read this. You may be a medical professional, seeking more insight into the patient. You may currently be a patient trying to seek answers in a difficult time. Or you may be a family member, partner, or friend of someone who is going through this challenging journey and trying to find ways to support them. I hope that sharing my story shed some light, gave some food for thought or, at least, provided some starting points.

Looking back, I realize that I started finding a lot of answers, when I became more courageous and formed my own opinion again, instead of being frozen in fear. Whoever you are and for whatever reason you came to read this book, I wish you have a strong voice in your own healing process.

And thank you, my proofreaders: Ann Cameron, Hester Kuipers, David Silke and Milia Chan.

List of Creams

> *Note*
> Do not apply any creams or products onto your skin before you go to your radiotherapy sessions unless your doctor agrees.

This is a list of creams that worked for me during and after the treatment and I do not receive any benefits from the manufacturers.

Most of the creams and remedies below share some similarity in their mode of action, like being moisturizing and/or help with itchy skin. However, each of them worked for me in different situations during my journey. You will need to find out for yourself which ones do the trick best in acute moments for you.

Make sure you take care of the skin in the radiotherapy field. Your skin will be very sensitive after a few weeks of radiotherapy until some weeks after the therapy ends.

> *Some general advice (from learning my lesson):*
> - Don't use soap in the area treated, just wash with warm water.
> - Try to avoid any extremes of temperatures, such as hot water during showering for example.
> - Don't use hot warming bottles nor cold packs on the treated area.
> - Be careful when drying your skin after showering and don't rub with the towel.
> - Use cream at least twice a day. Towards the end of my treatment and some weeks after there were days I put on creams/ointments even hourly.
> - Make sure you avoid direct sunlight on the treated skin as it will be very sensitive.
> - I would further recommend not to go swimming or to the sauna during therapy as this puts extra stress on the skin.

At some point, the vaginal mucosa was so irritated, sore and started itching like crazy. Some creams above helped but often not consistently. Another remedy that helped (when other creams failed) was a simple over-the-counter antifungal vaginal cream which then calmed the itching. Since this cream is typically used for a different purpose, I only used it only when nothing else seemed to help.

After the therapy had ended, I still developed (to this day) tiny wounds at the anus sometimes, especially when I eat for example lots of nuts and seeds. The skin is now just more fragile than it was before. When this happens, it makes it quite uncomfortable going to the toilet due to a burning feeling. What works for me quite well is to put on some lidocaine cream, which is a local anesthetic cream for which you can easily get a prescription from your GP.

The cream causes a temporary loss of feeling in the skin where it is applied onto. When I have these "burning issues", I sometimes also mix lidocaine with some Bepanthen cream and then apply it. This usually does the trick, calms the sharp pain, and accelerates the healing process.

Aquaphor ointment
Helps with dry/itchy skin in the radiation area.

Bepanthen creme
Provides intensive moisturization, especially in very dry and raw parts of the skin, gives relief, releases tension, and softens the skin. This was one of my favorite creams and I used it from some point every time after going to the toilet to provide a thick layer of cream to prevent urine getting to the open parts.

Red Relief
These are sterile gel dressing patches for burn wounds that help relieve the pain of skin areas that are open.

Weleda Sage Gums Balm
Preventative usage to protect gums during chemo.

Tannolact sitzbad
Calming and supports wound healing.

Eucerin AtopiControl
This cream is usually targeted at skin issues like Psoriasis, atopic Dermatitis but it helped me with itching of the radiated skin.

Again Life
This company has a whole series of products aimed at supporting cancer patients during and after the treatment period and also help with some chemo side effects on the skin. They have a whole series of products, the ones that I used were:
GutLife Creme - for inflamed anal mucosa,
EvaLife - for inflamed and itchy vaginal mucosa,
OraLife - for inflamed mouth mucosa.

Flamigel
This is a gel for treating low-grade radiotherapy-induced skin reactions like red, dry, itching, flaking, peeling or just irritated skin.

Silicea Gel
Has multiple uses. Mainly, I used it as cooling wound dressing, it calms the skin, eases pain, and helps with itching.

Engels Pluksel (Ointment dressing used here in the Netherlands)
This is simply medical fabric rolled up, which can be cut into the required sizes, applied with ointment, and then placed directly onto the wound, so that it "sticky - connects". Make sure you have this type of fabric for wound dressing on your hands. You cannot use Band-Aids on the radiated skin as it might take off a thin layer of skin when you remove it.

Dr Kade Hydrogel
Helps to treat dryness of the vagina and the adjacent intimate area and helps with itching, burning, sore feeling and skin irritation. This moisturizing gel is based on hyaluronic acid and is hormone free. I still use it almost every day.

Deumavan
This ointment helps with pain, itching, and dryness. It can help prevent infections and supports healing of skin conditions in the genital area, skin damage in the genital, anal area, and dry skin.

Useful links

AIN
Information on Anal intraepithelial neoplasia (AIN), what it is, staging & treatment options:
tinyurl.com/4sxpkc4d

General Information
The Anal Cancer Foundation and HPV Cancer Alliance pages provide in my view the most comprehensive informative pages around anal cancer:
www.analcancerfoundation.org
hpvca.org

Below is the guide (*Broschuere_Stoma_0620_LAYOUT3*) that I mentioned in previous chapters providing an overview of creams and remedies that could be used during and after adiotherapy. Please note the guide is only available in German:
tinyurl.com/wvujz8jh

Nutrition
Inflammation and cancer: Why your diet is important
An article on how inflammation might relate to cancer. Discussing long-term inflammation, how it can harm healthy cells and raise cancer risk. It further provides some information on how one can lower inflammation by making healthier lifestyle choices.
tinyurl.com/rfuevt8n

The inflammatory potential of diet in determining cancer risk; A prospective investigation of two dietary pattern scores
tinyurl.com/mrynfz8x

Nutrition, inflammation and cancer
www.nature.com/articles/ni.3754

The Power of Phytochemicals Combination in Cancer Chemoprevention
This article focuses on bioactive phytochemicals and their effect on cancer cells. With over 14 million new cases and approximately 8 million deaths annually, cancer is a global concern. The rise in mortality rates is due to tumor recurrence from treatment resistance, emphasizing the need for effective alternative management strategies. Phytochemicals have been identified for their ability to target various signaling molecules involved in cellular growth, proliferation, differentiation, and death, providing potential preventive strategies against cancer.
tinyurl.com/4s6n6a3j

Flavonoids as promising molecules in the cancer therapy: An insight
As cancer mortality rises, so does resistance to synthetic drugs, prompting the search for newer treatments. Phytochemicals, drawing from plant-based medicine, offer promising alternatives to current therapies. Challenges such as toxicity, resistance, and cost could be addressed by these compounds, particularly flavonoids, which have shown potential in modulating immune responses and inducing cell death. However, issues like bioavailability and drug interactions remain, requiring advanced techniques like nanotechnology. Understanding their mechanisms could lead to the development of cancer preventive drugs.
tinyurl.com/ycx3ccvf

And for carrots
Check this article, for example, at the National Library of Medicine:
Therapeutic Potential of Luteolin on Cancer – PMC
tinyurl.com/mwbf9zjb
Conclusion: "Luteolin has potent anticancer properties and is a natural substance that fights cancer in different ways. It helps control cell growth, regulates cell cycles, encourages cell death, and stops the formation of new blood vessels that feed tumors. When used together with traditional chemotherapy, it boosts its effectiveness. Combining luteolin with other similar substances makes it even more potent against cancer cells. Given its natural origin, Luteolin presents a promising avenue for new therapeutic approaches, potentially mitigating the toxicity associated with conventional chemotherapy."

Or, from the European Community Research and Development Information Service (CORDIS):
Raw carrots help prevent colon cancer, say Danish researchers
tinyurl.com/mumvsjpr
Researchers suggest raw carrots can help prevent colon cancer. The Danish Institute of Agricultural Sciences is trying to develop methods for growing carrots with higher levels of falcarinol. "Colon cancer is the second most common cancer in the EU, and there is currently no cure once it has become symptomatic, so testing and early detection are crucial."

Luteolin, a Potent Anticancer Compound: From Chemistry to Cellular Interactions and Synergetic Perspectives
tinyurl.com/2wkadtdr
This article discusses how luteolin could be a strong candidate for designing anticancer drugs as it is a natural compound that reduces inflammation, slows down cancer cell growth and encourages cancer cell death. Luteolin can also enhance the effectiveness of traditional chemotherapy when used together.

Links on Medical Mushrooms:

Immune Modulation From Five Major Mushrooms: Application to Integrative Oncology
This review looks at how five major mushrooms—Agaricus, Cordyceps, Reishi, Turkey Tail, and Maitake—affect the immune system in cancer treatment. It focuses on how these mushrooms change certain immune proteins in cancer models, their direct effects on cancer cells, and how they interact with chemotherapy drugs, affecting both their effectiveness and the side effects it causes. There's plenty of evidence from lab studies showing how these mushrooms fight cancer through the immune system, and early human studies show promise for treatment.
tinyurl.com/45fpxj2s

Medicinal Mushrooms (PDQ®)–Patient Version
Medical mushrooms have been used in Asia for centuries to treat infections, lung diseases, and cancer. In Japan and China, they are approved as part of cancer treatment, alone or with radiation or

chemotherapy. Over 100 types of mushrooms are used, including Reishi, turkey tail, shiitake, and maitake.

Researchers are studying how mushrooms boost the immune system and fight tumors. Compounds like betaglucans in turkey tail mushrooms may help. This summary focuses on Turkey Tail and Reishi mushrooms, covering how they're taken, what studies show, results from human trials, side effects, and FDA information.
tinyurl.com/579m5jje

Another article that focuses on which mushrooms might help to fight cancer is *What Is the Best Mushroom to Fight Cancer?*
tinyurl.com/ysb842ya

An article on the potential health benefits of turkey tail mushrooms, *Do turkey tail mushrooms benefit health?*
tinyurl.com/2nr8r963

Chaga mushroom: a super-fungus with countless facets and untapped potential
tinyurl.com/bdd4b62k

Using Chaga for Cancer: Here's What We Know
tinyurl.com/56h9sdtt

AHCC to treat HPV

Currently, there's no effective medicine or supplement for clearing high-risk human papillomavirus (HR-HPV) infections. This study looked at whether AHCC could help. The goal was to see if AHCC could boost the immune system to clear HRHPV infections. Conclusion: Both lab and animal studies showed lasting clearance of HPV infections.

From Bench to Bedside: Evaluation of AHCC Supplementation to Modulate the Host Immunity to Clear High-Risk Human Papillomavirus Infections
tinyurl.com/wu46mdf6
And similar results here:
AHCC® Supplementation to Support Immune Function to Clear Persistent Human Papillomavirus Infections
tinyurl.com/2p8eyy7f

Articles on fasting

Intermittent Fasting and Cancer
Fasting reduced side effects such as fatigue, weakness, and gastrointestinal complications. This study supports the concept that fasting is safe during chemotherapy, that it reduces some adverse effects, and that it does not interfere with the therapeutic effect intended.

Effect of fasting therapy in chemotherapy-protection and tumor-suppression: a systematic review
tinyurl.com/ysh6zhxx
Overall, fasting was found to have considerable effects in reducing chemotherapy side-effects (organ damage, toxic features, immunosuppression, reduced body weight and chemotherapy-induced death), suppressing tumor progression (tumor growth, metastasis, metabolic activity), and improving survival. Besides, fasting duration of longer than 48 hours was found to be crucial for exerting the effects of fasting therapy.

Treatment options to address side effects after therapy (as well possible if you had prior a hormone sensitive tumor):

Vaginal laser therapy
Vaginal laser therapy is a minimally invasive, non-surgical, nonhormonal procedure that stimulates new collagen production for healthier tissue. The laser delivers controlled heat energy to the vaginal tissues, which stimulates collagen production, increases blood flow, and supports tissue regeneration. This procedure can be used to address issues such as vaginal dryness, itching, burning, pain during intercourse, vaginal laxity (looseness), urinary incontinence, and some symptoms of menopause.

This treatment also gives women with a history of estrogen-dependent tumors a treatment choice as it seems to produce comparable results to Vaginal Estrogen Therapy!
Vaginal Laser Therapy Comparable to Vaginal Estrogen Therapy for Genitourinary Syndrome of Menopause
tinyurl.com/53sxuhb3

Effect of the Fractional CO2 Laser on the Quality-of-Life General Health, and Genitourinary Symptoms in Postmenopausal Women With Vaginal Atrophy: A Prospective Cohort
After menopause, women may experience vaginal atrophy due to hormonal changes. This study evaluated the effect of fractional CO2 laser treatment on the quality of life, vaginal atrophy symptoms, and urinary incontinence. The treatment significantly improved quality of life, sexual satisfaction, and reduced urinary incontinence symptoms.
tinyurl.com/v68kamba

Fractional Co2 laser for vulva-vaginal atrophy in gynecologic cancer patients: A valid therapeutic choice? A systematic review
This article discusses that CO2 laser therapy may be a novel, non-estrogen option to ease menopausal symptoms for women. Preserving quality of life after cancer therapy and managing menopausal symptoms are significant challenges for gynecological cancer survivors and also gynecologists. The article lists further references.
tinyurl.com/25m59h8m

PRP Treatment
Autologous Platelet-Released Growth Factor and Sexual Dysfunction Amendment: A Pilot Clinical Trial of Successful Improvement Sexual Dysfunction after Pelvic Irradiation
PRP (platelet-rich plasma) therapy can be used to treat various body parts and has been used in sports medicine for many years to address tendon, ligament, muscle, and/or cartilage injuries. This involves drawing blood, centrifuging it to produce PRP, and then injecting it back into the body to harness its own healing capacity. This article discusses its positive impact on sexual dysfunction after pelvic radiotherapy.
tinyurl.com/36s3yd4k

Platelet-rich plasma (PRP) for the treatment of chronic rectal ulcer: A case report – (about a patient who had chemoradiation)
This article discusses a patient with a history of rectal cancer and chemoradiation who experienced bloody stool for over 4 months. Various medications were tried, with limited success, and the rectal ulcer remained unhealed. The ulcer nearly healed within 9 days after

two PRP treatments.
tinyurl.com/52p85vk4
Minimally Invasive Treatment of Recurrent Anal Fistulas with Autologous Platelet-Rich Plasma Combined With Internal Orifice Closure.
This article explores the use of PRP as a minimally invasive procedure for treating anal fistulas, as it can accelerate the healing process of "challenging wounds", such as anal fistulas which also can occur after radiotherapy.
tinyurl.com/5n6vy78x

Cancer trials
Your hospital and/or doctor will have information on available trials, however if you would like to search through national and international trial databases you find some links here:
International: www.clinicaltrials.gov
US specific:
www.cancer.gov/research/participate/clinical-trialssearch

Work and Cancer Macmillian PDF
This is a great booklet for anyone who is working and has been diagnosed with cancer. It provides guidance for employed individuals as well as for employers and managers on how to support and deal with the situation. Additionally, this booklet contains great information for family members, friends and carers for people affected by cancer.
tinyurl.com/3ch8ebct

HRT Related Links
A critique of Women's Health Initiative Studies (2002-2006)
The article suggests that the WHI study made mistakes in its conclusions due to not adjusting for certain factors. Critics say the study wasn't properly randomized, and the women in it were already past menopause (and past the golden window mentioned in chapter 6). Hormone therapy should start earlier for prevention. Despite this, the study claimed hormone treatment increased risks, causing confusion and potentially denying women beneficial therapy.
tinyurl.com/4kywa9fz

The Controversial History of Hormone Replacement Therapy
This article covers the powerful effects of HRT on postmenopausal symptoms before unfortunately, the publication of the WHI trial abruptly stopped HRT use, even though evidence of harm was inconclusive. Further studies indicate HRT is beneficial for symptomatic women within 10 years of menopause or under 60. Despite its potential benefits, low HRT use continues globally.
tinyurl.com/42asfuxa

Glossary

AIN Anal intraepithelial neoplasia (AIN) indicates that there are abnormal cells in the lining of the anus. Another name for AIN is anal squamous intraepithelial lesions (SILs). This name refers to the type of cells impacted, because most of the abnormal cells are so-called squamous cells which make up the middle and outer layers of the skin. AIN is not cancer, but the cells might develop into cancer in the future. As for cancer, staging is used to capture how severe the cell changes are. *(See AIN staging Chapter 1, see Anal Cancer staging Chapter 5)*

Angiogenesis is the process of forming new blood vessels.

Apoptosis is the process when cells naturally self-destruct in the body.

Bioidentical Hormones are substances created from plant sources but are created synthetically. Bio-identical does not stand for "**organic**" but suggests that the body identifies them as very similar or equal to the body's own hormones. The related therapy is called BHRT (Bioidentical Hormone Replacement Therapy). Products of conventional HRT (Hormone Replacement Therapy) are usually prepared from the urine of pregnant horses and synthetically produced hormones.

Biopsy is a procedure to remove a small tissue sample from suspicious areas, which will then be sent for further microscopic investigation to the laboratory.

Cell proliferation is the process by which cells grow and divide. Uncontrolled cell division and unregulated cell death underlies almost all cancers.

Chemotherapy is a medication-based treatment that uses powerful chemicals to attack fast-growing cells in the body. It can be administered intravenously or as tablets. Chemotherapy is mostly used to treat cancer, as cancer cells grow and multiply out of proportion and much faster than healthy cells in the body.

There are more than 100 different chemotherapy drugs available. Some of them are used as standalone, others in combination to treat a variety of cancers. Though chemotherapy is an effective way to treat many kinds of cancer, it is still a toxic treatment and therefore carries the risk of side effects. Some chemotherapy side effects are mild and treatable, while others can cause serious complications.

Chemotherapy can be used in different ways, for example, to cure cancer as the primary or even sole treatment. It can be used after treatments, to attack hidden cancer cells. For instance, after surgery, to kill any cancer cells that might remain in the body. This is called adjuvant therapy. Another type of chemotherapy is to prepare for other treatments, for example, to shrink a tumor to make surgery and/or radiotherapy possible. This is called *neoadjuvant therapy*. Chemotherapy can further be used to ease symptoms of cancer by killing some of the cancer cells. This is called *palliative chemotherapy*.

Colonoscopy is a procedure during which a doctor checks the inside of the entire colon or large intestine. For the procedure, a long flexible tube is used which is called a colonoscope. The tube has a light and a tiny camera on one end. It is placed in the rectum and then moved up into the colon. This procedure allows the examination of the lining of the colon and rectum.

CT-scan (computed tomography) scan is an imaging procedure that uses a combination of X-rays and computer technology to produce images of the inside of the body. Most of the time IV (intravenous) contrast agent is used in the procedure. CTs can show detailed images of any part of the body, including the bones, muscles, fat, organs, and blood vessels. Important to understand is that CTs can create a picture of a larger area, for example, of the complete torso.

Flavonoids are phytochemical compounds present in many plants, fruits, vegetables, and leaves. They have potential applications in medicinal chemistry. Flavonoids possess a number of medicinal benefits, including anticancer, antioxidant, anti-inflammatory, and antiviral properties.

HPV stands for human papillomavirus, a very common group of viruses that affect the skin. There are more than 100 types of human papillomaviruses and they usually do not cause any problems in people. However, some types can cause issues like genital warts or even cancer.

Immunotherapy is a treatment method that uses the immune systems to fight cancer and autoimmune disorders. Unlike chemotherapy, which directly targets cancer cells, immunotherapy boosts the body's natural defenses to recognize and eliminate cancer cells or regulate autoimmune responses. There are various types of immunotherapies that enhance the immune response in distinct ways.

Boosting immune response: helping the immune system to recognize and attack abnormal cells like cancer. Cancer cells can hide from the immune system, but immunotherapy activates or improves the immune response to target them.

Blocking immune checkpoints: Some immunotherapies block molecules that cancer cells use to avoid immune attacks. By blocking these, immunotherapy allows the immune system to recognize and destroy cancer cells.

CAR T-cell therapy: T-cells are part of the immune system and develop from stem cells in the bone marrow. They help the body to protect against infection and even in fighting cancer. In this therapy CAR T-cells are created by taking T-cells from the patient and changing them in a lab to have special proteins on their surface called chimeric antigen receptors (CARs). These CARs can find and attach to specific proteins, called antigens, on cancer cells.

Monoclonal antibodies are lab-made antibodies that can stick to cancer cells, marking them for destruction by the immune system or blocking their growth.

Cytokines are proteins that help regulate the immune response. They can be used in immunotherapy to boost the immune system's ability to target cancer cells.

Cancer vaccines work like traditional vaccines, training the immune system to recognize and attack cancer cells. They contain substances found in cancer cells to trigger an immune response. Some cancer vaccines are even personalized to a person's individual's tumor. These vaccines are made using antigens derived from the patient's own tumor cells to increase the chances to trigger a targeted immune response.

Immunotherapy has shown promise in treating various cancers like melanoma, lung cancer, kidney cancer, lymphoma, and leukemia, as well as managing autoimmune diseases like rheumatoid arthritis and multiple sclerosis. However, it can have side effects as well such as fatigue, skin rash, diarrhea, and inflammation. Some patients might get more serious immune-related side effects that require close monitoring. Despite potential side effects, immunotherapy represents a significant advancement in treatment options to improve outcomes for patients with cancer and other diseases.

Lymph nodes are small, bean-shaped structures that are part of the body's immune system. These nodes are scattered throughout the body, but concentrated in areas such as the neck, armpits, groin, and abdomen. Lymph nodes filter, trap and destroy bacteria, viruses, and abnormal cells, including cancer cells, that may be circulating in the lymphatic fluid.

Lymph nodes are crucial in cancer diagnosis, staging and treatment, guiding decisions by indicating the extent of cancer spread (metastasis). In cases like lymphoma or melanoma for example, doctors may perform procedures to remove affected lymph nodes.

Cleaning or removing lymph nodes can help prevent cancer spread and guide treatment decisions, but they also carry potential risks like infection, lymphedema (swelling due to lymph fluid buildup), and impaired immune function. The decision to perform lymph node removal needs to be carefully considered in conversation with doctors and consultation with the patient, considering both the potential benefits and risks.

Micronutrients include vitamins and minerals.

Macronutrients include carbohydrates, proteins, and fat.

Menopause is a natural biological process that marks the end of a woman's menstrual cycles. It defines the moment after a woman has gone twelve months without a menstrual period. There is no set time for when menopause will happen, and it can occur when women are in their 40s or 50s, but in the Western world, the average age is 51 years. Menopause is the transition from fertile to infertile state.

MRI Magnetic Resonance Imaging (MRI), is a non-invasive medical imaging technique used to produce detailed images of the internal structures of the body. It uses a strong magnetic field and radio waves to generate images of organs, tissues, and other bodily structures. MRIs are used to zoom in on specific organs or areas in the body to get an exact image.

PET scan Positron emission tomography (PET) scans produce detailed 3D pictures of the inside of the body. A small amount of radioactive glucose (a type of sugar, a natural carbohydrate) is injected into a vein. This is based on the theory that tumor cells take up more glucose than normal cells. The PET scanner rotates around the body and captures where the glucose is being used. Tumor cells show up brighter in the picture than normal cells.

Perimenopause is the time leading towards menopause. It is a natural process triggered when a woman's ovaries gradually stop working. Ovulation may become inconsistent at first and then stop. The length of the menstrual cycle might become irregular before a woman has her final period. Symptoms that can accompany peri-menopause are caused by the changing levels of hormones in the body.

Phytochemicals are chemical compounds produced by plants to help them resist fungi, bacteria, and virus infections, as well as consumption by insects and other animals. This is one of the defense mechanisms of plants.

Post menopause marks the period that follows the menopause, twelve months after a woman had her last period. During this stage, women develop a higher risk for certain diseases due to the change in hormone levels. Further women might have/continue to have postmenopausal symptoms like hot flashes, irritability, mood swings, insomnia, dry vagina, difficulty concentrating, stress incontinence, urge incontinence, depression and more.

Proctoscopy is a procedure to examine the rectum and anus using a lighted tube called a proctoscope. This examination is used to find tumors, reasons for bleeding, inflammation, or hemorrhoids.

Proton Therapy is a type of radiation therapy used in the treatment of cancer. It delivers targeted radiation to cancerous tumors with high precision, minimizing damage to surrounding healthy tissues. Unlike regular radiation therapy, which uses X-rays or photons to deliver radiation, proton therapy uses protons, which are positively charged particles.

Proton Therapy is more precise than other types of radiation therapy, and doctors can design radiation beams that exactly fit the shape and depth of the tumor! The proton beams then deliver most of their energy to the targeted tissue only. Currently, there are trials running tests for anal cancer patients to reduce treatment toxicity.

Radiation Therapy is a type of cancer treatment that uses ionizing radiation to kill cancer cells or stop them from growing and dividing. It can be used as a primary treatment for cancer or together with other treatments such as surgery or chemotherapy, or as palliative care to relieve symptoms and improve quality of life in advanced cancer cases. There are mainly two types of Radiation Therapy:

- External Beam Radiation Therapy (EBRT) is the most common form of radiation therapy, where a machine placed outside the body delivers the radiation beams directly to the tumor. This is a localized treatment which means it targets a specific part of the body.
- Internal Radiation Therapy (Brachytherapy) uses radioactive implants placed inside the body (temporarily or permanently) and in or near the tumor, delivering a higher radiation dose. Permanent implants release radioactivity that fades over time.

The side effects of radiation therapy vary depending on which part of the body is being treated, how high the radiation dose is, and of course the individual's overall health. Common side effects during treatment include fatigue, skin changes, nausea, and changes in appetite. Many side effects are temporary, but there can be some long-term side effects depending on the area, like, for example, the abdomen and pelvis.

Sigmoidoscopy is a procedure to check the sigmoid colon, which is the lower part of the colon/large intestine and close to the rectum and anus. It is carried out with a thin tube with a small camera and light inserted in the bum to check for abnormalities.

STD stands for sexually transmitted diseases that are transmitted via STIs, sexually transmitted infections. They're mainly spread through sexual contact and can be caused by bacteria, viruses, or parasites, passing from person to person in bodily fluids.

Stoma is an opening in the abdominal wall that a surgeon makes for waste to leave the body, with an exchangeable bag attached to it. A stoma can be but does not have to be permanent.

About the author

Leila Schwarz, born in Germany, shares her home in Amsterdam, The Netherlands, with her charming dachshund Archimedes. With over 20 years of experience in the technology sector, Leila currently holds a leadership role in an American tech company. She has built her career in a still predominantly male-driven industry with resilience and determination, leveraging her expertise to drive innovation and change.

Printed in Dunstable, United Kingdom